Atlas of Alzheimer's Disease

Atlas of Alzheimer's Disease

Edited by

Howard H Feldman MD FRCP(C)

Professor and Head, Division of Neurology,
Department of Medicine, University of British Columbia
and
Director, UBC Hospital Clinic for Alzheimer's Disease and Related Disorders,
Vancouver, British Columbia, Canada

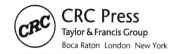

CRC Press
Taylor & Francis Group
Boca Raton London New York

CRC Press is an imprint of the
Taylor & Francis Group, an **informa** business

First published 2007 by Infroma UK Ltd

Published 2019 by CRC Press
Taylor & Francis Group
6000 Broken Sound Parkway NW, Suite 300
Boca Raton, FL 33487-2742

© 2007 by Taylor & Francis Group, LLC
CRC Press is an imprint of Taylor & Francis Group, an Informa business

First issued in paeprback 2019

No claim to original U.S. Government works

ISBN 13: 978-0-367-45298-8 (pbk)
ISBN 13: 978-0-415-39045-3 (hbk)

Visit the Taylor & Francis Web site at
http://www.taylorandfrancis.com

and the CRC Press Web site at
http://www.crcpress.com

A CIP record for this book is available from the British Library.
Library of Congress Cataloging-in-Publication Data

Composition by Exeter Premedia Services Private Ltd., Chennai, India

Dedication

This book is dedicated to all of the patients, and families that we have served at the UBC Hospital Clinic for Alzheimer's Disease and Related Disorders for the past 25 years. It has been your inspiration that continually motivates us to advance our research and clinical acumen that we may provide ever better care to you.

The authors also express their appreciation to all of the current and past staff at the Clinic for their helpful support and collaborations over many years.

The editor gratefully acknowledges the support of his wife Gail and his children Ben and Samantha without whose understanding and patience this book would certainly have not been possible.

Contents

List of contributors   ix

Foreword   xi
Serge Gauthier

Preface   xiii

1. Historical concepts of Alzheimer's disease and dementia   1
   Jacob Grand and Howard H Feldman

2. Epidemiology of Alzheimer's disease and dementia   27
   Ging-Yuek Robin Hsiung

3. The diagnosis of Alzheimer's disease and dementia   41
   Najeeb Qadi and Howard H Feldman

4. Pathophysiology of Alzheimer's disease   59
   Najeeb Qadi, Sina Alipour, and B Lynn Beattie

5. Neuropathology of Alzheimer's disease   71
   Ian RA Mackenzie

6. Prevention of Alzheimer's disease   83
   Claudia Jacova, Benita Mudge, and Michael Woodward

7. Treatment of Alzheimer's disease   105
   Najeeb Qadi, Michele Assaly, and Philip E Lee

8. Alzheimer's disease: the future   125
   Joyce Lin H Yeo and Howard H Feldman

Index   137

Contributors

Sina Alipour BSc
Research Assistant, Division of Neurology, Department of Medicine, University of British Columbia, Vancouver, BC, Canada

Michele Assaly MA
Research Coordinator, UBC Hospital Clinic for Alzheimer's Disease and Related Disorders, Vancouver, BC, Canada

B Lynn Beattie MD FRCP(C)
Professor Emeritus, Division of Geriatric Medicine, Department of Medicine, University of British Columbia; and UBC Hospital Clinic for Alzheimer's Disease and Related Disorders, Vancouver, BC, Canada

Howard H Feldman MD FRCP(C)
Professor and Head, Division of Neurology, Department of Medicine, University of British Columbia; and, Director, UBC Hospital Clinic for Alzheimer's Disease and Related Disorders, Vancouver, BC, Canada

Jacob Grand BSc
Research Assistant, Division of Neurology, Department of Medicine, University of British Columbia, Vancouver, BC, Canada

Ging-Yuek Robin Hsiung MD MHSc FRCP(C)
Assistant Professor, Division of Neurology, Department of Medicine, University of British Columbia and Providence Health Care, Vancouver, BC, Canada

Claudia Jacova PhD
Assistant Professor, Division of Neurology, Department of Medicine, University of British Columbia, Vancouver, BC, Canada

Philip E Lee MD FRCP(C)
Assistant Professor, Division of Geriatric Medicine, Department of Medicine, University of British Columbia; and Providence Health Care, Vancouver, BC, Canada

Ian RA Mackenzie MD FRCP(C)
Professor, Department of Pathology, Vancouver General Hospital, University of British Columbia, Vancouver, BC, Canada

Benita Mudge BSc
Research Coordinator, UBC Hospital Clinic for Alzheimer's Disease and Related Disorders, UBC Hospital, Vancouver, BC, Canada

Najeeb Qadi MD
Clinical Fellow, Division of Neurology, Department of Medicine, University of British Columbia, Vancouver, BC, Canada

Michael Woodward MD
Associate Professor, Director, Aged Care Services, Austin Health, University of Melbourne, Melbourne, Australia

Joyce Lin H Yeo MD
Clinical Research Fellow, Division of Neurology, Department of Medicine, University of British Columbia, Vancouver, BC, Canada

Foreword

In our current era of rapid progress in our understanding of Alzheimer's disease (AD), it is useful to look back at the two millenia of description of senescence, one century of the clinical and pathological characterization of AD, and thirty years of recognition of the cholinergic deficit that lead to the first symptomatic drugs for this condition. In addition to an accurate and detailed historical perspective, the authors of the 'Atlas of Alzheimer's Disease' are providing a state-of-the-art review of current working hypothesis, diagnostic approaches and treatments of AD. The many tables and illustrations help understand the scientific information provided and may facilitate knowledge transfer to all persons interested in AD. The next edition of this Atlas will hopefully include a description of safe and effective disease-modifying treatments for persons at genetic risk, persons in prodromal stages and persons in early stages of AD.

Serge Gauthier MD FRCPC
Professor, Departments of Neurology and
Neurosurgery, Psychiatry, Medicine,
McGill University,
Director, Alzheimer and Related Disorders
Research Unit,
McGill Center for Studies in Aging, Douglas Hospital,
Montreal,
Quebec, Canada

Preface

The publication of this Atlas of Alzheimer's Disease coincides with the 100th anniversary of Dr. Alois Alzheimer's presentation of the clinical and neuropathological findings of his patient Auguste D, during a lecture at the 37th Conference of South-West German Psychiatrists in Tübingen, Germany. His landmark findings heralded the first modern scientific recognition of the disease that bears his name. In reading the case description of Auguste D, one cannot help but experience the sense of helplessness that seemed likely to have engulfed the patient, her family and Dr. Alzheimer himself.

As this book will attest, the last 20 years have brought unprecedented new knowledge to our understanding of this disease and for the first time approved symptomatic treatments. This progress heralds the long awaited translation of benefit from neuroscience research, renewing the belief that continued progress will continue to change the face of this disease. We can foresee that this disease will become a chronic but manageable illness through many of its phases. It is with the goal of describing the progress and the great anticipation of imminent advances that my coauthors and I have prepared this monograph. Within the Atlas we start with the history of dementia as we have been able to track it across millennia, thereby setting the stage for the evolution of our more refined understanding of the last century. We then follow with chapters on the epidemiology, diagnosis, pathophysiology, and neuropathology. Finally, we conclude with a review of disease prevention and a futuristic vision of where we believe we are headed with Alzheimer's disease.

This book is published at a time when the demographics are changing in both industrialized and developing societies, when there is an unprecedented growth in our elderly population and in turn in individuals affected by Alzheimer's disease. In parallel to this exponential growth arises is an increasing demand for information. Our aim within this book is to provide a variety of audiences with the most up to date information presented in an accessible format with an emphasis on visual images. We hope that this Atlas format will provide medical professionals, other health care providers as well as families and patients with a source of useful and comprehensible information. We have emphasized the transitions of knowledge from the past through the present and to the future to allow the full picture to be seen within the largest possible perspective.

In 1982, the University of British Columbia Hospital opened its doors to the Clinic for Alzheimer's Disease and Related Disorders. Over the past 25 years this multidisciplinary clinic has provided assessment and care to an estimated 15,000 patients and families. The authors of this book have been affiliated with the Clinic in various capacities and collectively reflect many of the hard learned lessons, successes and challenges that we have faced. I am grateful for each of the authors contributions and salute them for this. Most of all we thank all of the patients that we are privileged to serve and whose lives we hope to improve in some meaningful way as they face Alzheimer's disease or related conditions.

Howard H Feldman

CHAPTER 1

Historical concepts of Alzheimer's disease and dementia
Jacob Grand and Howard H Feldman

INTRODUCTION

Alzheimer's disease (AD), the most common cause of dementia in the elderly, is a progressive neurodegenerative illness characterized by a spectrum of clinical features and neuropathologic findings. In the one hundred years since Dr Alois Alzheimer (Figure 1.1) first described the disease, considerable advances have been made in understanding the pathogenesis, epidemiology, diagnosis, and treatment of AD. The following chapter presents a broad historical framework of the evolution of both dementia and AD. The examination of the historical milestones of discovery which have culminated in the current definitions provides an important reminder that, what is new is sometimes old and what is old often renews.

ORIGINS OF DEMENTIA: GRECO-ROMAN PERIOD TO THE 19TH CENTURY

Greco-Roman period

The concept of dementia has evolved over 2500 years, from a vague notion of inevitable age-related cognitive impairment, to a contemporary understanding of its distinct clinical and pathologic features. The Greco-Roman model, 'senescence itself is an illness' (*senectus ipsa morbus est*), is frequently cited in ancient texts depicting mental decline as a natural consequence of aging.[1] One of the earliest references to age-related cognitive impairment is attributed to Pythagoras (582–507 BC), the Greek physician of the 7th century BC. Pythagoras divided the life cycle into five distinct stages, the last two of which

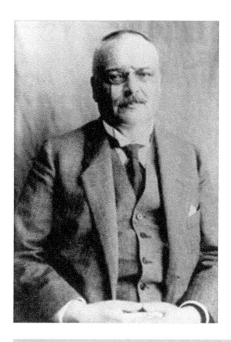

Figure 1.1 Dr Alois Alzheimer (1864–1915) Reproduced with permission of the Wellcome Library, London, UK.

were designated the *senium*, or 'old age'. These were periods of decline and decay of the body with a regression of mental capacities where 'The system returns to the imbecility of the first epoch of infancy'.[2] Hippocrates (460–377 BC), the father of medicine, attributed all illnesses to an imbalance in the four basic body fluids, or humors (blood, phlegm, yellow bile, and black bile). According to his Hippocratic theory, four primary and opposite fundamental qualities (hot, cold, wet, and dry) were associated with each of the humors. Mental decline was considered an inevitable consequence of aging, due to the associated imbalance of fluids, thus rendering the body 'cold' and 'dry'. Aristotle (384–322 BC) adopted a similar perspective, reasoning that old age is inseparable from cognitive decline. In support of his theory of aging, Aristotle advocated that elderly individuals should not be appointed high administrative posts within the government because 'They are gradually blunted by mental deterioration and can hardly fulfill their function'.[3] The Roman physician Galen (150–200 AD) systematized Greco-Roman medical knowledge, emphasizing the Hippocratic model of the brain's importance, as opposed to Aristotle's belief that the heart was the source of life and the seat of human cognition. Galen's writings included a diagnostic classification for dementia, or 'morosis', in his list of mental disorders and cited old age as a situation in which it occurred. Through the works of Pythagoras, Hippocrates, Aristotle, and Galen (Figure 1.2), it is evident that age-related cognitive decline was recognized as early as the 7th century BC, that in the Greco-Roman period mental deterioration was considered an inevitable consequence of aging, and that aging itself was considered a disease process.

The Middle Ages

The historic observations and commentary about aging and dementia greatly diminished following the collapse of the Greco-Roman empire in the 4th and 5th centuries AD. This paralleled the decline in all empirical research and scientific study in this era where theocracy ruled. Theological doctrines prohibited any heretical learning through observation and research, with the religious authorities of the time asserting that disease was a punishment for sin. In spite of the prevailing views, Roger Bacon (1214–1294), a Franciscan friar (Figure 1.3), promoted the use of experimentation to determine truth and advocated empiricism as a fundamental principle of

scientific investigation.[1] His defiance resulted in imprisonment, though while in solitary confinement Bacon completed his work, *Methods of Preventing the Appearance of Senility*. In this report he references the brain as the source of memory and cognition, rather than the accepted belief of the heart's dominance in emotion and all mental processes. Bacon proposed a 'ventricular system' with memory stored in the posterior ventricle, thought and judgment deriving from the middle ventricle, and imagination originating in the anterior ventricle.[4] There was no fundamental shift away from the continued perception that dementia was an inevitable feature of aging. There was, however, a surge of interest in dementia during the widespread persecution of witches in the 1400–1500s. Victims of witch trials undoubtedly included individuals with cognitive disorders. During this period there was little elucidation of the underlying causes of dementia, and diagnosis was based primarily upon the presence or absence of fever.

The 17th–19th centuries

The 17th century brought a better characterization of behavior and cognition, and their biologic basis. Dissection of the human body became accepted, and there was consequently an increased interest and capacity to characterize the physiologic changes in the brain that underlie mental disorders.[2] In 1664, Thomas Willis (1621–1675), the personal physician to King Charles II (Figure 1.3), coined the term neurology to mean 'the doctrine of the nerves' in his landmark book *Cerebri Anatome: Cui Accessit Nervorum Descriptio et Usus*. In Willis' *London Practice of Physick* (1685), he offered a comprehensive classification of dementias, recognizing that some people 'become by degrees dull, by the mere declining of age'. He further identified a number of causes of dementia including congenital factors, head injury, alcohol and drug abuse, prolonged epilepsy, disease, and old age.[2] Towards the end of the 18th century, examination of the brain and nervous system extended beyond anatomists and entered the realm of pathologists. Novel pathologic theories, based upon disturbed nervous function, replaced those of Hippocrates and Aristotle. In 1776, William Cullen (1710–1790) (Figure 1.3) reorganized all disease into four classes. It is in Cullen's classification, under Neuroses, that senile dementia (*Amentia senilis*) is recognized for the first time as a medical entity, defined as 'decay of perception and memory, in old age'.[5]

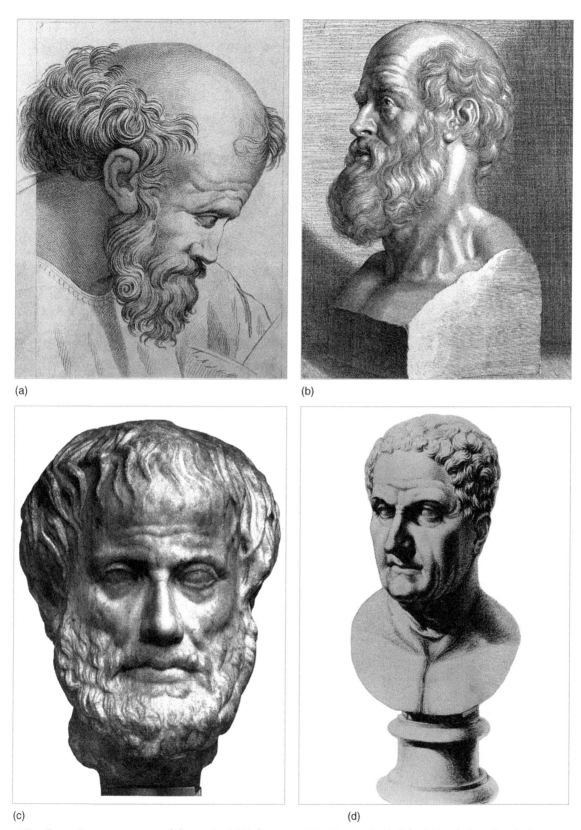

(a)

(b)

(c)

(d)

Figure 1.2 Greco-Roman concepts of dementia. (a) Pythagoras (569–475 BC) divided the life cycle into five distinct stages, the last two of which were designated the *senium*. Reproduced with permission of the Wellcome Library, London, UK. (b) Hippocrates (460–377 BC) considered mental decline an inevitable consequence of aging. Reproduced with permission of the Wellcome Library, London, UK. (c) Aristotle (384–322 BC) considered old age inseparable from cognitive decline. Reproduced with permission of the Wellcome Library, London, UK. (d) Galen (150–200 BC) systematized concepts of Greco-Roman medical knowledge, including a diagnostic classification for dementia (*morosis*). Reproduced with permission of the Wellcome Library, London, UK.

(a)

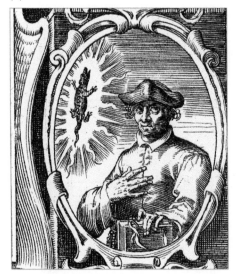

(b)

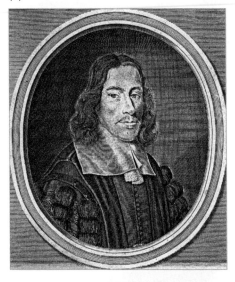

(c)

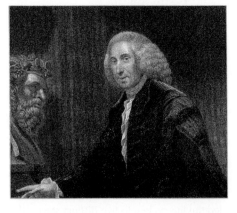

Figure 1.3 The Middle Ages and 17th–19th century concepts of dementia. (a) Roger Bacon (1214–1294) published *Methods of Preventing the Appearance of Senility* in which he references the brain as the source of memory and cognition, and proposes a 'ventricular system'. Reproduced with permission of the Wellcome Library, London, UK. (b) Tomas Willis (1621–1675) coined the term *neurology* as the 'Doctrine of the Nerves' in 1664. Reproduced with permission of the Wellcome Library, London, UK. (c) William Cullen (1710–1790) categorized all disease into four classes in 1776, including senile dementia (*Amentia senilis*) under the classification of neuroses. Reproduced with permission of the Wellcome Library, London, UK.

At the turn of the 19th century a series of pivotal developments in the progress of mental disorders, including senile dementia, occurred. The first major steps were implemented by the French physician Phillippe Pinel (1745–1826) at the Bicêtre asylum in Paris (Figure 1.4). In his 1806 book *Treatise on Insanity*, Pinel advocated the development of institutions for humane and appropriate care of mentally ill individuals. Pinel promoted the

(a)

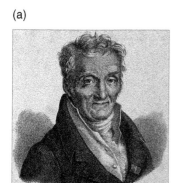

(b)

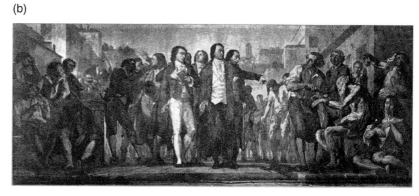

Figure 1.4 Phillippe Pinel (1745–1826) implemented numerous humanitarian reforms at the Bicêtre asylum in Paris. Pinel's 1806 publication, *A Treatise on Insanity*, promoted humane and appropriate care for individuals with mental disorders. (a) Phillipe Pinel. Reproduced with permission of the Wellcome Library, London, UK. (b) Phillipe Pinel at the Bicêtre asylum in Paris. Reproduced with permission of the Mary Evans Picture Library, UK.

application of scientific principles of objective observation in clinical settings. Furthermore, Pinel's endorsement of humanitarian reforms encouraged widespread clinical and pathologic observations of a variety of mental disorders. One of Pinel's students, Jean Etienne Esquirol (1772–1840) (Figure 1.5), recognized the need to establish a revised classification system of mental disorders. Esquirol's 1838 publication, *Des Maladies Mentales*, introduced detailed descriptions of newly identified subtypes and categories of mental disorders. One such refinement was the fundamental distinction between dementia and amentia, where dementia is 'the loss of mental faculties consequent on disease'. He characterized amentia not as a disease, but as a 'condition in which the intellectual faculties are never manifested; or have never developed sufficiently to enable the individual to acquire knowledge'. Esquirol presented a number of possible causes of dementia, reflecting the accepted medical opinions of the mid-19th century.[4]

After Pinel and Esquirol had laid the groundwork for systematic observation and description, it became possible to recognize detailed characteristics of mental disorders. The application and practice of differential diagnosis resulted in the emergence of senile dementia as a more defined condition. By the end of the 19th century new concepts and techniques established the basis for an etiologic characterization of mental disorders. In 1864, Sir Samuel Wilks (1824–1911) (Figure 1.6) provided a definitive description of atrophy and changes in brain weight that accompanied some dementias, as well as aging.[2] Although the term arteriosclerosis was first used in 1833, it was not until the late-19th

century that pathologists came to view it as a prominent disease mechanism. Rudolf Virchow's (1821–1902) (Figure 1.6) concept of the pathogenesis of arteriosclerosis became a widely accepted model. He believed that vascular degeneration was important as a general cause of disease, and specifically was the principle cause of lesions associated with old age. In 1894, Otto Binswanger (1852–1929) (Figure 1.6) described a dementia caused by extensive arteriosclerotic demyelination of the subcortical white matter.[5]

At the same time that vascular disease became established as a predominant cause of senile dementia, improvements in microscopy and new histochemic techniques allowed elements of the nervous system to be visualized for the first time. In 1892, Gheorghe Marinescu (1863–1938), Paul Blocq (1860–1896), and Victor Babes (1854–1926) described a novel pathologic feature, the accumulation of an unidentified substance into plaques, in the brain of an elderly epileptic patient. In 1898, the same pathology under the name 'miliary sclerosis' was observed in two cases of senile dementia. The term 'miliary' comes from the Latin word for the grain millet and was used to describe lesions whose morphology had the shape and size of millet seeds (Figure 1.7).[3]

At the end of the 19th century dementia was considered a condition of cognitive and psychologic impairment associated with chronic brain disease. Early efforts were made to measure the symptoms and severity of dementia, to ascertain the differential importance of the senile and vascular etiologies of dementia, and to study the comparative prevalence of senile dementia in relation to other mental disorders affecting the elderly.

(a)

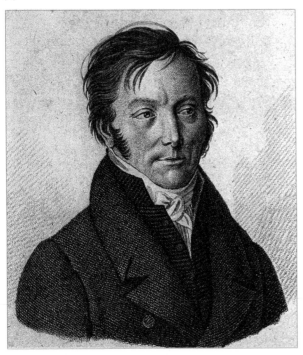

(b)

Head injuries	Mercury abuse
Progression of age	Wine abuse
Hemorrhoid surgery	Political upheavals
Sequelae of delivery	Unhappy love
Ataxic fever	Dietary excess
Syphilis	Masturbation
Paralysis	Unfulfilled love
Mania	Domestic problems
Apoplexy	Poverty
Menstrual disorders	Fears

Figure 1.5 Jean Etienne Esquirol (1772–1840) established a revised classification system of mental disorders in his 1838 publication, *Des Maladies Mentales*. Esquirol presented detailed descriptions of mental disorders, including the distinction between dementia and amentia. (a) Jean Etienne Esquirol. Reproduced with permission of the Wellcome Library, London, UK. (b) 19th Century causes of dementia.

TOWARDS A MODERN UNDERSTANDING OF ALZHEIMER'S DISEASE: THE 20TH CENTURY

1900–1930

Alois Alzheimer (1864–1915)

Alois Alzheimer (Figure 1.8) was born on 14 June, 1864, in Markbreit, a small town in southern Germany. Dr Alzheimer received his medical training from the Universities of Berlin, Tübingen, and Wurzburg, graduating in 1888 upon completion of his doctoral thesis, *On the ceruminal glands of the ear* (Figure 1.9). Alzheimer's research interests were wide ranging and included not only dementia of degenerative and vascular origin, but also psychoses, forensic psychiatry, and epilepsy. In 1889, Alzheimer began his training in neuropathology at the Stadische Irrenanstalt in Frankfurt, where he met and formed a long and creative partnership with Franz Nissl (1860–1919) (Figure 1.10).[5] While in

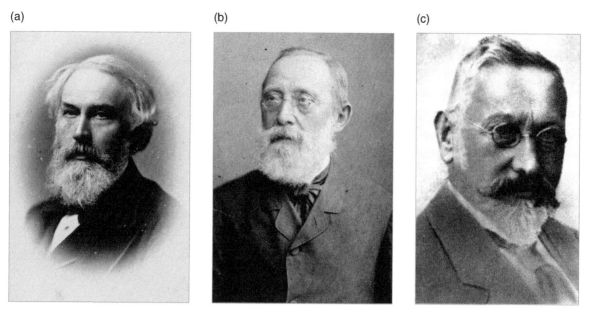

Figure 1.6 Late-19th century contributions to the etiologic characterization of dementia. (a) Samuel Wilks (1824–1911) provided a definitive description of atrophy and changes in brain weight associated with dementias. Reproduced with permission of the Wellcome Library, London, UK. (b) Rudolf Virchow's (1821–1902) concept of arteriosclerosis and vascular degeneration as the principle causes of age-related lesions became a widely accepted model. Reproduced with permission of the Wellcome Library, London, UK. (c) Otto Binswanger (1852–1929) described a dementia caused by extensive arteriosclerotic demyelination of the subcortical white matter in 1894.

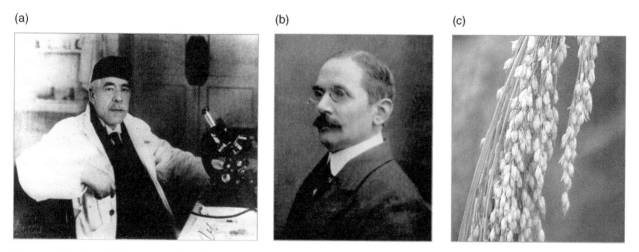

Figure 1.7 Late-19th century developments in microscopy and histology. In 1892, Gheorghe Marinescu (1863–1938) (a) and Victor Babes (1854–1926) (b) described a novel pathologic feature, the accumulation of an unidentified substance into plaques, or 'miliary sclerosis' (c). By 1898, this pathology was observed in numerous cases of senile dementia.

Frankfurt, Alzheimer expressed his belief that research and clinical practice should be combined as essential elements of scientific enquiry: 'Why should not the physician improve his competence by enlarging scientific knowledge besides doing his daily clinical practice?'.[4] Together, Alzheimer and Nissil developed and applied histologic stains, illuminating the cellular pathology of the brain to an unprecedented degree. Their reputations earned them invitations to join Emil Kraepelin (1856–1926) (Figure 1.10), the founder of modern psychiatry, in Heidelberg. While there, Kraepelin supervised Alzheimer's research on the histopathology of general paralysis of the insane. In 1894, Dr Alzheimer married Nathalie Geisenheimer (1860–1901) (Figure 1.8). Three children came from their marriage. In 1903, Dr Alzheimer joined Dr Kraepelin in Munich, where he

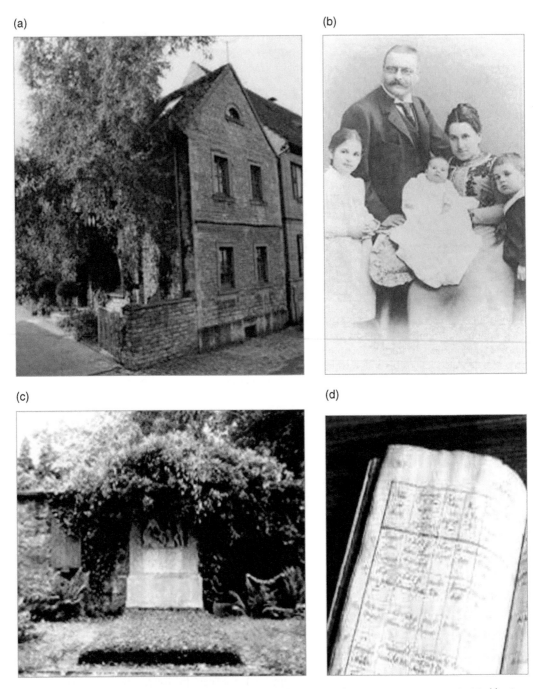

Figure 1.8 The life of Dr Alois Alzheimer (1864–1915). (a) Alois Alzheimer was born on 14 June, 1864, in Markbreit, a small town in southern Germany. (b) In 1894, Dr Alzheimer married Nathalie Geisenheimer (1860–1901). Three children came from their marriage. (c) At the age of 51 years, Dr Alzheimer developed a severe and persistent cold which developed into subacutre bacterial endocarditis. On 19 December, 1915 Alois Alzheimer died in a uremic coma. (d) Dr Alzheimer's personal notebook and signature.

was appointed head of the neuroanatomic laboratory for brain research (Figure 1.10). Alzheimer's lab achieved international acclaim, resulting in a large number of visiting psychiatrists and neuropathologists including Gaetano Perusini (Italy), Francesco Bonfiglio (Italy), Ugo Cerletti (Italy), Hans Gerhard Creutzfeldt (Germany), Alfons

Jakob (Germany), Karl Kleist (Germany), and Nicolas Achucarro (Spain).

In 1912, the Friedrich-Wilhelm University of Breslau appointed Dr Alzheimer as the Chair of the Department of Psychiatry and Director of the University Psychiatric Clinic (Figure 1.9). Dr Alzheimer viewed the appointment

(a)

(b)

(c)

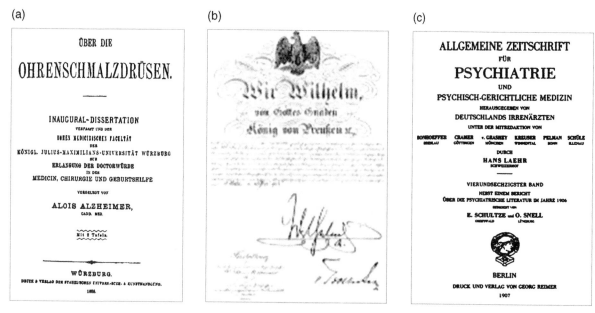

Figure 1.9 Dr Alzheimer's academic and professional achievements. (a) Alois Alzheimer's doctoral thesis from the University of Wurzburg (1888), *On the ceruminal glands of the ear.* Graeber MB (2004) Alois Alzheimer (1864–1915). International Brain Research Organization Neuroscience History. (b) Dr Alzheimer's appointment in 1912 as the Chair of the Department of Psychiatry at the Friedrich-Wilhelm University of Breslau. (c) On 3 November 1906 Dr Alzheimer presented the case of Auguste D at the 37th Conference of South-West German Psychiatrists in Tübingen, Germany. In 1907, Dr Alzheimer published his findings, *About a peculiar disease of the cerebral cortex.*

(a)

(b)

(c)

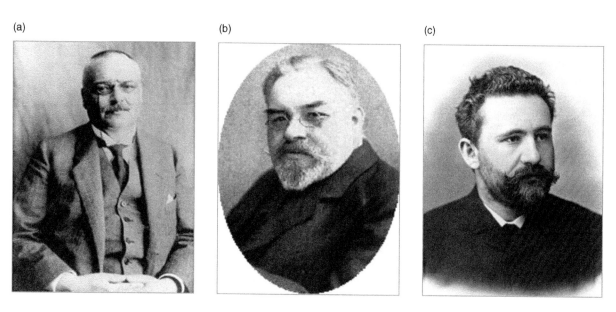

Continued...

as the fulfillment of his scientific and academic goals. On a trip returning to Breslau, Alzheimer developed a severe and persistent cold which developed into subacute bacterial endocarditis. He never recovered and on 19 December 1915 Alois Alzheimer died in a uremic coma.[2]

The First Case: Auguste D

At the turn of the 20th century, Max Bielschowsky (1869–1940), the German neuropathologist, improved

upon the silver stain (*reazione nera*) originally discovered by Camillo Golgi (1843–1926) in 1873, and for the first time made it possible to visualize cellular components of neurons (Figure 1.11). While previously, using a carmine stain, it was only possible to make glial elements visible, Bielschowsky identified threadlike structures within neurons which he called neurofibrils.[5] In 1906, using the Bielschowsky method, Dr Alzheimer described a startling new pathology in the brain of one of his

(d)

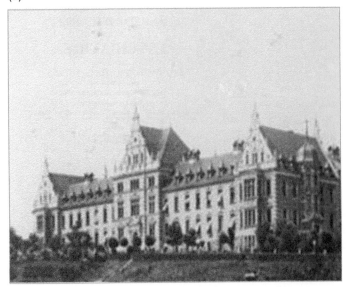

(e)

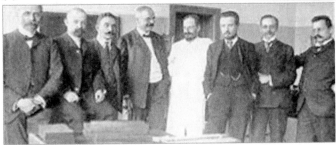

(f)

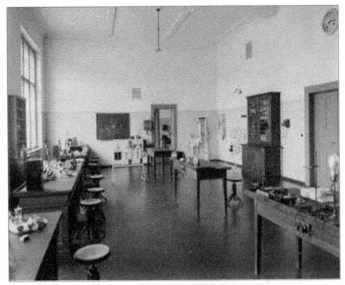

Figure 1.10 Dr Alzheimer's community. (a) Dr Alois Alzheimer. Reproduced with permission of the Wellcome Library, London, UK. (b) In 1889, Alzheimer began his training in neuropathology at the Stadische Irrenanstalt in Frankfurt, where he met and formed a long and creative partnership with Franz Nissl (1860–1919). (c) Emil Kraepelin supervised Alzheimer's research while at the Universities of Heidelberg and Munich. The eponym 'Alzheimer's disease' is attributed to Dr Kraepelin, who included the term in his 1910 publication, *Textbook of Psychiatry* (8th edn). (d) University of Tübingen, where Dr Alzheimer presented the case of Auguste D. (e) University of Munich (Royal Psychiatric Clinic). (f) Dr. Alzheimer's laboratory at the University of Munich.

patients. Auguste D, a 51-year-old woman, was first examined by Dr Alzheimer on 25 November 1901, when she was admitted to the Frankfurt Hospital (Figure 1.12). She presented with a striking cluster of clinical symptoms including progressive amnestic disorder, aphasia, alexia, and agraphia, accompanied by disorientation, unpredictable behavior, profound agitation, auditory hallucinations, paranoia, and pronounced psychosocial impairment.

(a)

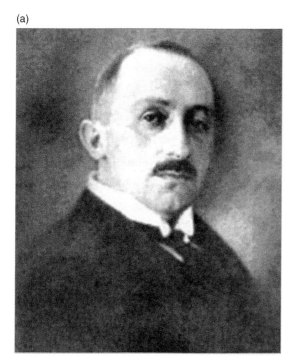

(c)

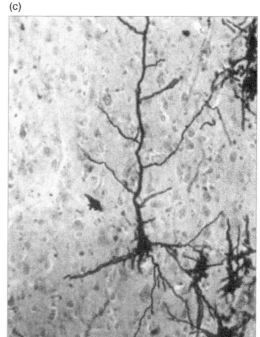

(b)

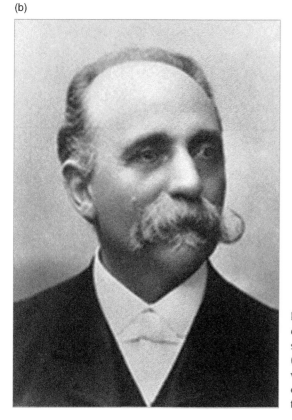

Figure 1.11 Early 20th century histology. At the turn of the 20th century, Max Bielschowsky (1869–1940). (a) improved upon the silver stain (*reazione nera*) originally discovered by Camillo Golgi (1843–1926). (b) in 1873, and for the first time made it possible to visualize cellular components of neurons. Reproduced with permission of the Wellcome Library, London, UK. (c) Camillo Golgi's drawing of the hippocampus impregnated by his stain.

Auguste D died within four and a half years of the onset of symptoms, in April 1906.[6]

The rapidity of degeneration and relatively young age of the patient made this clinical course unusual, and prompted Dr Alzheimer to investigate the neuropathologic features. One quarter to one third of cerebral cortical neurons had disappeared, and many of the remaining neurons contained thick, coiled tangles of fibrils within their cytoplasm. Using the Bielschowsky silver method, Dr Alzheimer observed intense staining

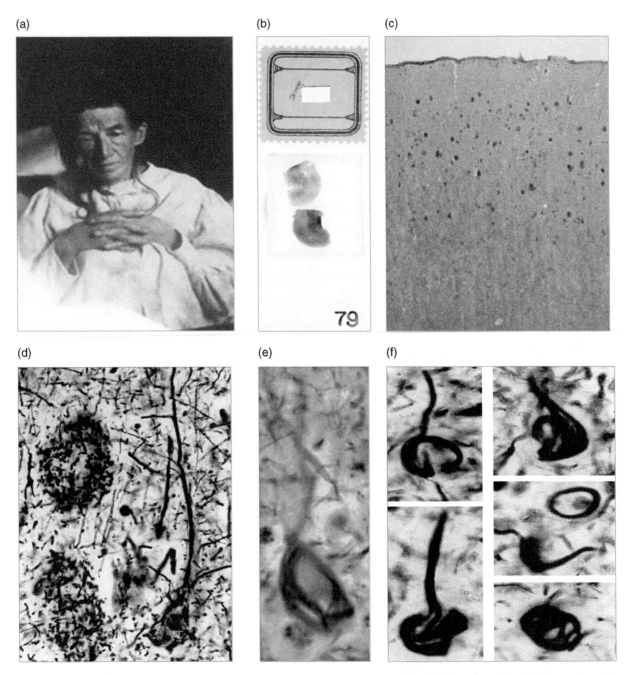

Figure 1.12 The first case: Auguste D (1906). (a) Auguste D (age 52 years). (b) Bielschowsky-stained tissue sections from Auguste D. (c) & (d) Bielschowsky-stained amyloid plaques from Auguste D. (e) & (f) Bielschowsky-stained neurofibrillary tangles from Auguste D.

of the neurofibrils and speculated that a chemical change had occurred. Furthermore, Dr Alzheimer suggested that the fibrils led to the eventual death of the cells, leaving the 'tangle' as a marker of cell death. In addition to the stained neurofibrillary tangles and accompanying neuronal degeneration, Dr Alzheimer noted the widespread presence of plaque pathology matching the original description of 'miliary sclerosis' by Marinescu et al in 1898.[2]

The clinical and neuropathologic presentation of Auguste D stood out quite distinctly against the background of dementias Dr Alzheimer had studied, most often being neurosyphilis and vascular disease. The young age of dementia onset, the unusual clinical picture, including the rapidity of progressive decline, coupled to the neuropathology and the severity and types of lesions, extended outside of the available nosologic framework of mental disorders. On 3 November 1906 Alzheimer presented the case of Auguste D at the 37th Conference of South-West German Psychiatrists in Tubingen, Germany, in a lecture entitled *On the peculiar disease process of the cerebral cortex* (Figure 1.9). In the following year, Alzheimer published his findings under the title *About a peculiar disease of the cerebral cortex*.[7] In 1907, Fischer presented a detailed report on the histopathologic changes in dementia, and in 1908 Bonfiglio described a patient, aged 60 years, who displayed similar symptoms and neuropathology to the case of Auguste D. In 1909, Gaetano Perusini (1879–1915) a friend and colleague of Alzheimer, investigated four cases including that of Auguste D in his paper, *On histological and clinical findings of some psychiatric diseases of older people*. Perusini presented detailed histopathologic findings with illustrations depicting amyloid plaques and neurofibrillary tangles. In summary he stated, 'The pathological process re-calls main features of senile dementia; however, the alterations in the cases described are more far reaching, although some of them represent presenile dementia'.[8]

The eponym Alzheimer's disease

Following these seminal descriptions of Dr Alzheimer and his colleagues, pathologists began to consider the condition a unique disease entity, often referencing the condition as 'Alzheimer's disease'.[9] Official endorsement of the eponym is attributed to Dr Emil Kraepelin who included the term 'Alzheimer's disease' in his 1910 publication, *Textbook of Psychiatry* (8th edn).[7] Kraepelin described Alzheimer's disease as a special subtype of senile dementia – presenile dementia – stating that 'The clinical interpretation of this Alzheimer's disease is still unclear'. Although the anatomic findings suggest that this condition deals with an especially severe form of senile dementia, the fact that this disease may arise even at the end of the fifth decade does not allow this supposition. In such cases we should at least assume a 'senium praecox' if not perhaps a more or less age-independent unique disease process.[5]

In addition to his analysis of presenile dementia on a histologic level, Kraepelin's behavioral observations capture many of the basic features and neuropsychiatric changes associated with the disease, 'In most cases, the psychological alterations of old-age result in the disease pattern of dementia. The main features consist of a gradually developing psychological weakness, in which there exists a decrease in receptivity, decrease of mental resilience, restriction of sentimental relationships,

slackening of energy, and the development of obstinate unmanageability'. Kraepelin described details of the types of memory impairments associated with the disease, commenting that 'Past events gradually vanish from their memory, although often events of their childhood are recalled in their mind with surprising vividness. Moreover, acquired abilities also gradually fail; the patient forgets foreign languages, cannot remember names or numbers, and fails in mathematical problems. In particular the memory of recent events starts to reveal numerous and incomprehensible gaps'.[2]

In 1911, following Kraepelin's naming of the disease, Dr Alzheimer published a further comprehensive report of his conceptualization of the disease. This paper included a re-examination of Auguste D, along with a detailed description of a second case of dementia. Johann F, a 56-year-old man was admitted to Alzheimer's psychiatric clinic in Munich on 12 November, 1907: 'In the previous 6 months he had become forgetful, lost the ability to perform normal daily tasks, and developed prominent agnostic, aphasic, and apractic disturbances'. After 3 years of hospitalization, Johann F died on 3 October 1910. Neuropathologic examination revealed the widespread presence of amyloid plaques, but not a single neuron showing neurofibrillary tangles in the cerebral cortex. Alzheimer identified Johann F as a case of 'plaque-only' pathology (Figure 1.13).[10]

1910–1930

The great burst of initial enthusiasm following Alzheimer's initial discoveries and Kraepelin's naming of the disease promptly dissipated over the following two decades. Alzheimer's disease received very little attention in the scientific literature and much was left unresolved by 1930. There was uncertainty about the relationship of senile dementia to normal aging, and considerable confusion regarding the classification of AD as a distinct disease entity. Researchers could not agree about the relative importance of cerebral arteriosclerosis as a cause of senile dementia. There was no agreement as to whether arteriosclerosis and the Alzheimer-type neuropathologic changes were related to one another.[11]

1930–1980

Over the next half-century pathologic techniques evolved to include histochemical and cytochemical approaches,

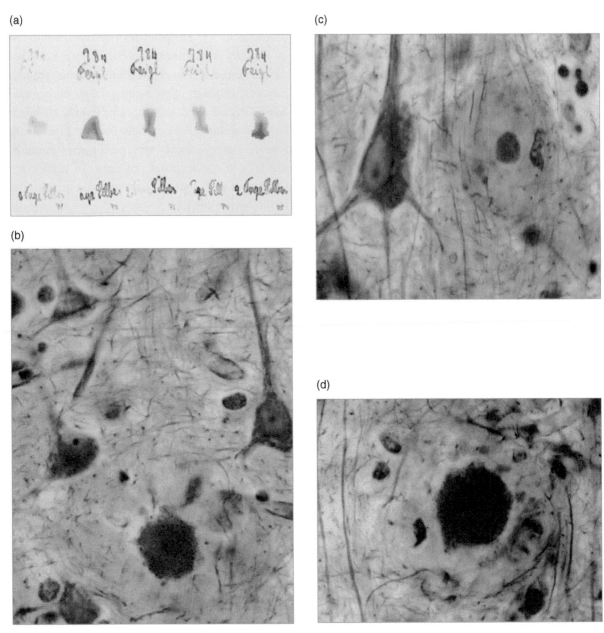

Figure 1.13 The second case: Johann F (1911). (a) Bielschowsky-stained tissue sections from Johann F. (b)–(d) Cerebral cortex Bielschowsky-stained amyloid plaques from Johann F.

as well as ultrastructural studies. These were applied to research investigations of plaques and tangles with productive outcomes. However, the central issues of contention during these decades concerned the validity of AD as a separate disease category from senile dementia, whether AD was truly the cause of dementia in the elderly, and if normal senescence or cerebral arteriosclerosis was responsible for cognitive impairments in older persons. In 1948, Newton and later Neuman and Cohn (1953) suggested that the clinical presentations of 'pre-senile' and 'senile' dementia were identical forms of the disease.[12]

It was not until 1955, when Roth demonstrated that mental changes could be caused by a variety of both functional and organic diseases, that the modern era of knowledge about AD and dementia began. Today, it is recognized that dementia is a symptom complex that has many possible causes and diseases to which it may be associated. The challenge of distinguishing brain changes resulting from healthy aging began in a number of landmark studies by Blessed, Tomlinson, and Roth in the mid-1960s. In order to settle the uncertainty of AD etiology, clarification around the contributions of the clinical, biologic, and neuropathologic aspects of the disease was required. Such comparisons became possible in the early 1960s with the introduction of the electron microscope (EM) as a research tool and the development of quantitative measures of dementia.

In the early 1960s, Terry et al (US) and Kidd et al (UK) reported the finding of EM studies showing that the ultrastructure of a neurofibrillary tangle contains masses of fibers with a periodic structure. These were established to be paired helical filaments (PHF) (Figure 1.14). These findings enabled the field to develop quantitative assessments of these hallmark lesions, to further define the ultrastructure of the amyloid core (neuritic plaque), and to develop methods of isolating plaques, neurofibrillary tangles, and PHFs.

These early ultrastructural investigations clearly set the stage for the discovery of more sophisticated molecular and immunologic probes to further characterize the molecular neurobiology of AD.[13]

In 1968 and 1970 Tomlinson, Blessed, and Roth proposed an instrument to objectively evaluate aspects of cognition, function, and behavior in AD. Their prospective studies then correlated quantitative measures of dementia with estimates of the number of lesions (plaques), and the volume of brain atrophy. Tomlinson et al established that the types of lesions that characterize and cause dementia are also present in the brains of many non-demented elderly individuals. Consequently, clinical distinctions between the two groups rested largely upon the quantity of pathology

(a)

(b)

(c)

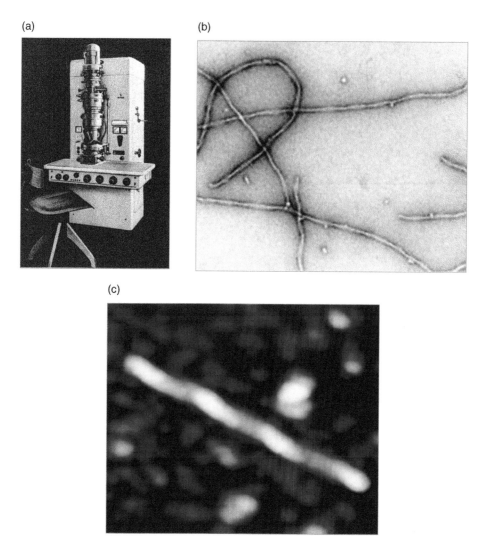

Figure 1.14 Ultrastructural studies of AD pathology. (a) Electron microscope (EM). In the early 1960s, EM studies demonstrated that the ultrastructure of a neurofibrillary tangle contains masses of fibers with a periodic structure. These were established to be paired helical filaments (PHFS). (b and c).

present, rather than its nature. These pioneering studies emphasized the importance of measurement in pathology and helped establish the quantitative boundaries for AD. Additionally, Tomlinson et al focused on the cumulative presence of ischemic (embolic) cortical infarctions as the cause of vascular dementia, playing down the role of small vessel arteriosclerosis with the white matter. They estimated that infarction of ≥100 cc of brain would almost be invariably associated with dementia (Figure 1.15). This led to the term 'multi-infarct dementia' (MID) as a pathologic entity.[14,15]

Systematic biochemical investigations of the brains of AD cases began in the mid- to late-1970s. The hope was that a clearly defined neurochemical abnormality would be identified, providing the basis for the development of rational therapeutic interventions. Support for this perspective came from numerous studies which reported substantial deficits in the enzyme responsible for the synthesis of acetylecholine (ACh), choline acetyltransferase (ChAT). Subsequent discoveries of reduced choline uptake, ACh release, and loss of cholinergic perikarya from the nucleus basalis of Meynert confirmed a substantial presynaptic cholinergic deficit. These studies, together with the emerging role of ACh in learning and memory, led to the 'Cholinergic hypothesis of Alzheimer disease' (Figure 1.16). It was proposed that degeneration of cholinergic neurons in the basal forebrain, and the associated loss of cholinergic neurotransmission in the cerebral cortex and other areas, contributed significantly to the deterioration in cognitive function seen in individuals with AD.[16]

THE CONTEMPORARY CHARACTERIZATION OF AD: 1980–PRESENT

The last several decades have marked an unprecedented new era of scientific progress in the field of AD, where the pace and breadth have surpassed the previous 100 years of investigation. As a result of this research progress, it is now possible to investigate AD biochemically, pathologically, and clinically. Central to the current understanding of the disease has been the progress in genetics, neuroimaging, diagnosis, and therapeutic interventions.

Genetics of AD

Genetic studies undertaken in the early 1980s began to elucidate patterns of autosomal dominant inheritance, as well as other evidence for genetic risk factors. Chromosome 21 attracted particular attention, firstly for its relationship to Down's syndrome (DS) given the extra chromosome (trisomy 21) (Figure 1.17a). In 1981, Heston et al reported that relatives of 125 subjects who had autopsy-confirmed AD exhibited a significant excess of dementia, consistent with genetic transmission. Compared to controls, the relatives of affected individuals were derived from families with a significantly greater incidence of DS (trisomy 21).[17] While this connection is still not fully explained, it is particularly noteworthy given the extremely high prevalence of AD neuropathology in the brains of middle-aged patients with DS.

In 1984, Glenner and Wong[18] reported the amino acid sequence of the main component of β-amyloid, a 4-kDa peptide termed 'amyloid beta protein' (Aβ) (Figure 1.17b). Subsequently, the gene encoding the amyloid precursor protein (APP) was isolated and mapped to chromosome 21[19] (Figure 1.17c). The discovery of autosomal dominant mutations in APP heralded numerous breakthroughs in the genetics of AD.

(a)

(b)

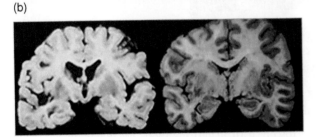

Figure 1.15 Volumetric brain changes in AD. (a and b) AD brain (left) vs normal brain (right).

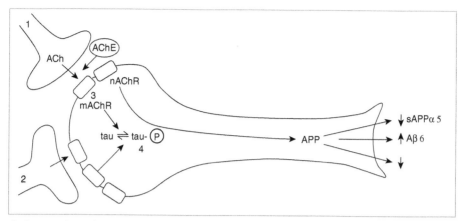

Figure 1.16 Cholinergic hypothesis of AD. Schematic diagram of a neuron representing alterations in neurotransmission in Alzheimer's disease: (1) reduced cortical cholinergic innervation; (2) reduced corticocortical glutamatergic neurotransmission due to neuron or synapse loss; (3) reduced coupling of muscarinic M1 receptors to second messenger system; (4) shift of tau to the hyperphosphoryalted state – precursor of neurofibrillary tangles; (5) reduced secretion of soluble APP; (6) increased production of β-amyloid protein; (7) decreased glutamate production.

This impacted not only the small number of identified families, but also the subsequent elucidation of the secretases which process APP and the β-amyloid core. In the mid-1990s genetic linkage studies uncovered mutations in presenilin 1 (PSEN1) on chromosome 14,[20] and presenilin 2 (PSEN2) on chromosome 1.[21] Presenilin forms the active site of the γ-secretase complex involved in the production of Aβ (Figure 1.17d). Cleavage of APP by γ- and β-secretases produces the Aβ peptide which aggregates into plaques (Figure 1.17e). To date, a total of 16 autosomal-dominant mutations of APP have been found, 140 in PSEN1 and 10 in PSEN2.[22]

During this period of molecular discovery, genetic risk factors for both familial and sporadic forms of AD were identified. Apolipoprotein E (ApoE) gene polymorphisms were shown to be involved in late-onset familial cases of AD. In particular, the ε4 allele of ApoE was found to be associated with an increased risk of developing AD.[23,24] ApoE can bind Aβ and localizes to senile plaques, supporting the theory that this protein plays a key role in the clearance of Aβ (Figure 1.17f).

To date, no mutations in the tau gene have been associated with familial AD. However, neurofibrillary tangle pathology appears to play an important role in AD progression. Mutations in the tau gene on chromosome 17 have been associated with the class of frontotemporal dementias with parkinsonism (FTDP-17). These tauopathies present with tau aggregations in neurons and glia, without any amyloid deposits, and produce a clinical phenotype of frontotemporal dementia (FTD) which is clinically distinguishable from AD.[25]

Amyloid cascade hypothesis

Major neurogenetic advances over the past two decades, including studies of cell- and animal-based model systems, have supported the development of the 'amyloid cascade hypothesis' (Figure 1.18). In 1991, it was suggested that accumulation of Aβ in the brain is the primary force driving AD pathogenesis, with the rest of the disease process resulting from an imbalance between Aβ production and Aβ clearance. Within the proposed cascade, the dysregulation in APP processing initiates the AD pathogenic events leading to aggregations of Aβ, specifically Aβ42. Formation of neuritic plaques instigates further pathologic events, including the formation of NFTs, disruption of synapses, reduction in neurotransmitters, death of tangle-bearing neurons, and an important inflammatory response.[26,27]

Since the initial identification of Aβ as the main component of amyloid plaques, evidence has accumulated that this peptide is indeed the inciting neuropathologic event in AD. Central to this hypothesis is the observation that the vast majority of mutations causing familial early-onset AD (EOAD) increases the ratio of fibrillogenic Aβ42.[22] In addition, transgenic mice models expressing pathogenic mutations of APP and PS1 have increased levels of Aβ and amyloid plaques.[28] Furthermore, individuals with trisomy 21 have three

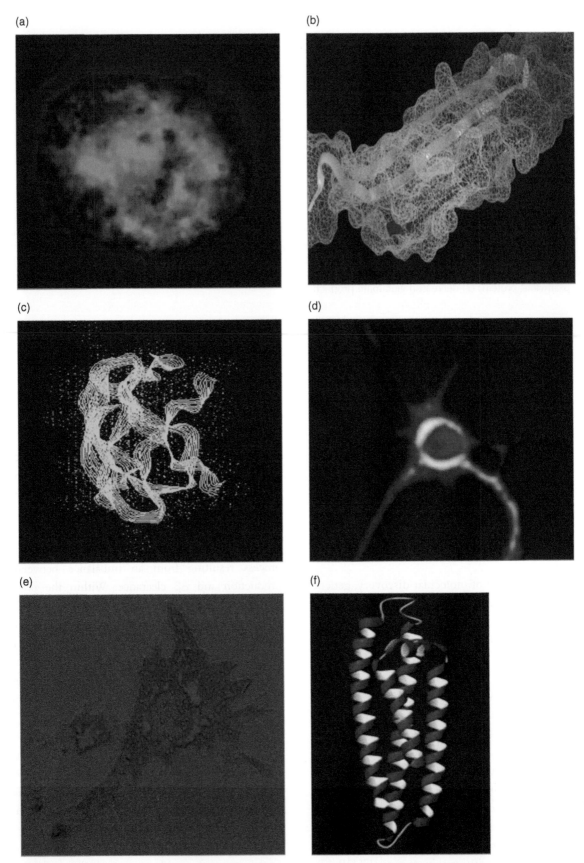

Figure 1.17 The genetics of AD. (a) Individual with trisomy 21 (Down's syndrome) exhibit high prevalence rates of AD neuropathology. (b) 'Amyloid beta protein' (Aβ), a 4-kDa peptide. (c) Amyloid precursor protein (APP). (d) Presenilin. (e) β-secretase. (f) Apolipoprotein E (ApoE).

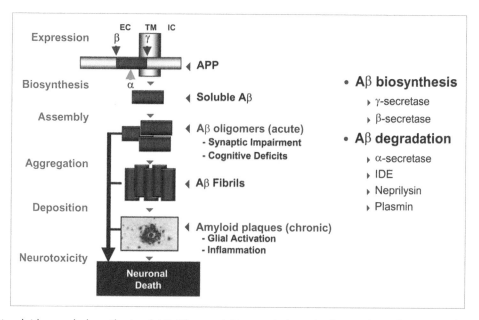

Figure 1.18 Amyloid cascade hypothesis of AD. The amyloid cascade hypothesis postulates that accumulation of Aβ in the brain is the primary force driving AD pathogenesis, with the rest of the disease process resulting from an imbalance between Aβ production and Aβ clearance.

copies of APP and develop advanced AD, usually within the fourth decade of life.

Consistent with the amyloid cascade hypothesis, large amounts of *in vitro* Aβ are neurotoxic to cells. Aβ exerts its neurotoxic effects in a variety of ways, including disruption of mitochondrial function, induction of apoptotic genes, formation of ion channels triggering loss of calcium homeostasis, stimulation of the JNK/SAPK pathway, activation of microglia cells leading to the expression of pro-inflammatory genes, an increase in reactive oxygen species, and eventual neuronal toxicity and death[29] (Figure 1.19).

Neuroimaging

Beyond the elucidation of the biochemical basis of AD, the last several decades have also witnessed major advancements in neuroimaging techniques. A range of methods have been developed which are both sensitive and specific to the anatomic and physiologic brain changes associated with AD (Figure 1.20). These methods include high-resolution structural imaging with computed tomography (CT) or magnetic resonance (MR), and functional neuroimaging techniques, such as single photon emission CT (SPECT), positron emission tomography (PET), and functional MRI (fMRI). In addition to their clinical applications for diagnosis, these techniques offer

the opportunity to examine structural, functional, and biochemical changes in the pathogenesis of AD.

The advent of CT scanning in the 1970s made visualization of the brain parenchyma possible for the first time. In the following decades, significant advances in hardware, computing power, and imaging programs have led to improved image resolution. In the 1980s, MR imaging was added, allowing higher resolution and novel scanning with greater visualization of gray and white matter, water diffusion, and other pathologic disturbances. CT and MR have matured to be routinely useful in clinical assessment. However, due to unresolved issues around sensitivity and specificity for the diagnosis of AD, they are primarily used adjunctively to assess the degree and pattern of atrophy and comorbid pathologies. In some instances, they allow for the identification of other specific causes of dementia including normal-pressure hydrocephalus, vascular dementia, or tumors.[30]

The development of PET techniques measuring metabolism and blood flow using radioactive ligands evolved during the 1970s. PET advances have led to breakthroughs in understanding cerebral blood flow, glucose metabolism, and neurotransmitter function in AD. PET scanning visualizes uptake of radioactive tracers, with the majority of studies using fluorodeoxyglucose (FDG), which is taken up by the glucose

(a)

(b)

(c)

(d)

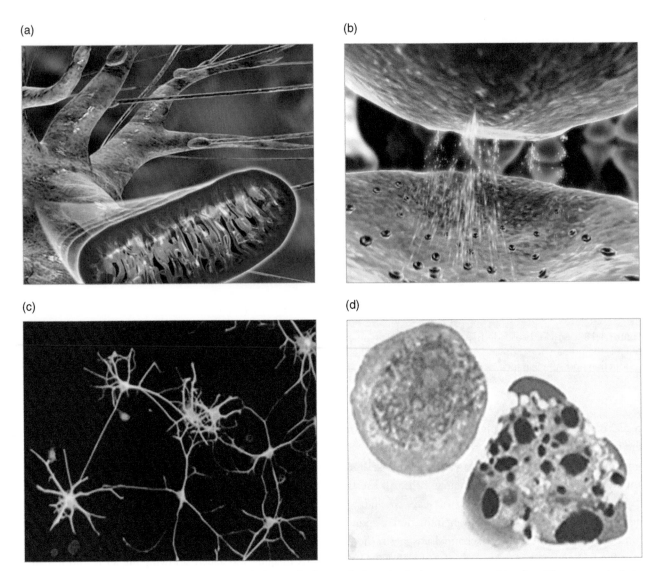

Figure 1.19 Aβ Neurotoxicity. Consistent with the amyloid cascade hypothesis, large amounts of *in vitro* Aβ are neurotoxic to cells. Aβ exerts its neurotoxic effects in a variety of ways, including disruption of mitochondrial function (a), induction of apoptotic genes, formation of ion channels (b), triggering loss of calcium homeostasis, stimulation of the JNK/SAPK pathway, activation of microglial cells (c), leading to the expression of pro-inflammatory genes, an increase in reactive oxygen species, and eventual neuronal toxicity and death (d).

transporter and reflects the brain's metabolic rate of glucose consumption. Many investigators have shown that AD is characterized by reduced FDG uptake in the temporal parietal cortex, especially the posterior cingulate gyrus and the medial temporal lobe. Recent developments in neuroimaging of AD have investigated the use of PET ligands for brain amyloid, including F19 2-dialkylamino-6-acylmalononitrile substituted naphthalenes (FDDNP) and the C11 Pittsburgh compound (PIB). PIB appears relatively specific for senile neuritic plaques (SNPs) in AD, while FDDNP likely binds SNPs and NFTs.[31,32] Since structural changes occur late in the course of AD, functional imaging modalities may

have greater potential in identifying subtle pathologic changes earlier during the course of the disease. In the 1990s, the development of fMRI allowed the study of cortical activation patterns, and more subtle changes in brain activation.[30]

Diagnosis

One of the most important advances in the contemporary study of AD has been the development and widespread adoption of diagnostic clinical criteria. The *Diagnostic and Statistical Manual of Mental Disorders*, third edition (DSM-III),[33] required that AD have 'a loss

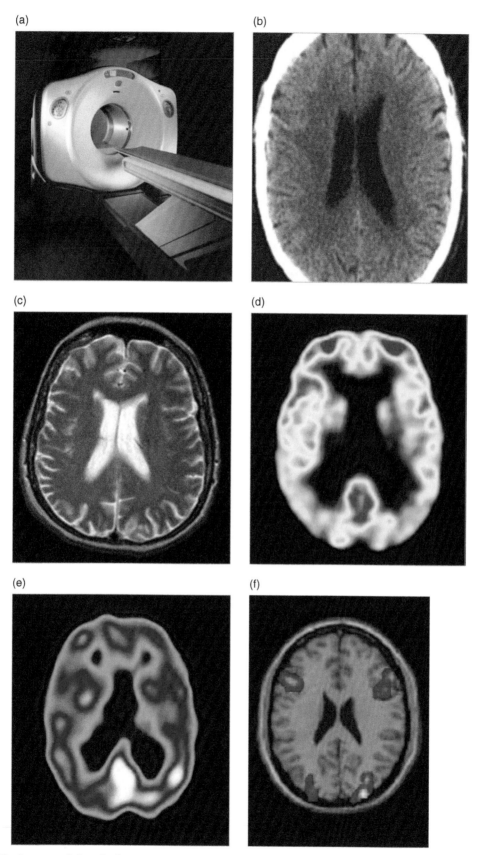

Figure 1.20 The last several decades have witnessed major advancements in neuroimaging techniques (a). A range of methods have been developed which are both sensitive and specific to the anatomic and physiologic brain changes associated with AD, including: (b) Computed tomography (CT), (c) magnetic resonance (MR), (d) positron emission tomography (PET), (e) single photon emission CT (SPECT), and (f) functional MRI (fMRI).

of intellectual abilities of sufficient severity to interfere with social or occupational functioning'. Subsequently, a greater degree of specification came through the National Institute of Neurological and Communicative Disorders and Stroke–Alzheimer's Disease and Related Disorders Association (NINCDS-ADRDA) diagnostic criteria in 1984,[34] and the *Archives of Neurology* report 'Diagnosis of Alzheimer's disease' in 1985.[35] The NINCDS-ADRDA criteria specified inclusion-exclusion factors, encompassing three levels of confidence: probable, possible, and definite. In 1997, the Khachaturian neuropathologic criteria were further advanced by the National Institute on Aging (NIA)–Reagan criteria.[36] These efforts have refined the clinical diagnostic descriptions of AD, facilitated the identification of clinical-pathologic correlations, assisted the development of objective measures of behavior-psychometric assessment, and established the infrastructure for longitudinal research studies.

In the past two decades, significant progress has been made in the standardization of these diagnostic criteria (reliability, sensitivity, specificity). Currently, AD is assessed using a variety of validated scales, including measures of:

(1) Cognition: Mini-Mental State Examination (MMSE);[37] Alzheimer's Disease Assessment Scale–cognitive subscale (ADAS-cog);[38] Activities of Daily Living (ADL);[39] Disability Assessment for Dementia (DAD).[40]

(2) Behavior: Neuropsychiatric Inventory (NPI);[41] Behavioral Pathology in Alzheimer's Disease Rating Scale (BEHAVE-AD).[42]

(3) Global functioning: Clinician's Interview-Based Impression of Change (CIBIC);[43] Clinical Dementia Rating Scale (CDR).[44]

These criteria have become the gold standard for diagnostic classification and provided the basis for clinical research in molecular biology, genetic analyses, and therapeutic interventions.

Treatment

The past decade has seen the first approved treatments for the symptoms of AD. Acetylcholinesterase inhibitors (AChEIs) became available for public use between 1993 and 2002. Memantine, an uncompetitive *N*-methyl-

D-aspartate (NMDA) receptor antagonist gained approval for AD from 2002 to 2006. This progress in symptomatic therapies heralded the first light of therapeutic hope, with disease modifying therapy still elusive.

Acetylcholinesterase inhibitors

The AChEIs inhibit synaptic acetylcholinesterase, the enzyme responsible for degrading acetylcholine, and aim to augment cholinergic neurotransmission (Figure 1.21a). The first use of AChEIs in AD dates back to 1979, when physostigmine was investigated.[45] Physostigmine did not present a favorable benefit–risk ratio for AD patients. Its acetylcholinesterase inhibition was limited, selectivity was poor, and penetration through the blood–brain barrier insufficient. However, these pioneering studies stimulated the successful development of the next generation of AChEIs, with markedly improved pharmacokinetic and pharmacodynamic profiles. Currently, four AChEIs (tacrine, donepezil, rivastigmine, and galantamine) are approved in most countries worldwide (Figure 1.21b–e).

The glutamatergic basis of AD therapy

Beyond cholinergic augmentation, glutamatergic neurotransmission is another symptomatic target in AD. Glutamate is the major excitatory neurotransmitter in the central nervous system and plays an important role in neurotransmission and plasticity. Glutamate-driven signaling is central to the process of long-term potentiation (LTP), a cellular mechanism that underlies learning and memory.[46,47] An increase of extracellular glutamate can lead to excessive activation of NMDA receptors and, consequently, intracellular calcium accumulation which can induce a secondary cascade resulting in neuronal death (Figure 1.22).

Memantine is a non-competitive, moderate-affinity, NMDA antagonist that protects neurons against glutamate-mediated excitotoxicity without preventing physiologic activation of the NMDA receptor.[48] Memantine was approved for the treatment of moderate to severe AD in 2002 by the European Agency for the Evaluation of Medical Products (EMEA), and in 2003 by the FDA (Figure 1.22).

Disease-modifying therapeutic strategies

The era of approved disease-modifying therapies for AD has not yet opened, but is being approached. Immunotherapeutic studies of Aβ vaccine, gamma secretase inhibitors or modulators, and amyloid

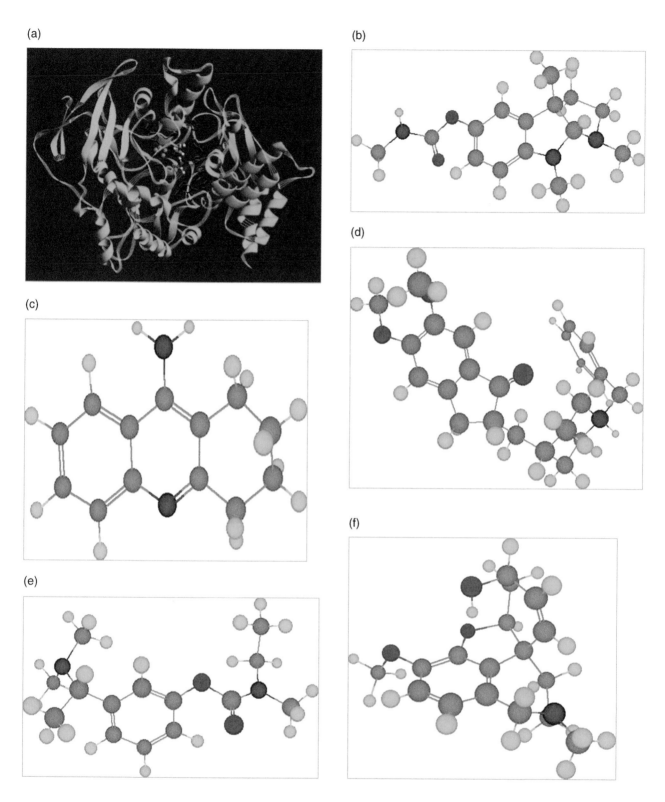

Figure 1.21 Treatment of AD. The past decade has seen the first approved treatments for the symptoms of AD. Acetylcholinesterase inhibitors (AChEIs) inhibit synaptic acetylcholinesterase (a), the enzyme responsible for degrading acetylcholine, and aim to augment cholinergic neurotransmission. First generation AChEIs include (b) physostigmine and (c) tacrine. Second generation AChEIs include (d) donepezil, (e) rivastigmine, and (f) galantamine.

(a)

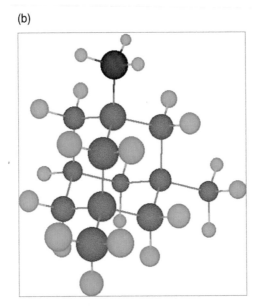

(b)

Figure 1.22 The glutamatergic basis of AD therapy. Glutamate is the major excitatory neurotransmitter in the central nervous system and plays an important role in neurotransmission and plasticity (a). An increase of extracellular glutamate can lead to excessive activation of N-methly-D-aspartate (NMDA) receptors and, consequently, intracellular calcium accumulation which can induce a secondary cascade resulting in neuronal death. Memantine (b) is a non-competitive, moderate-affinity, NMDA antagonist that protects neurons against glutamate-mediated excitotoxicity without preventing physiologic activation of the NMDA receptor.

anti-aggregants have all entered into clinical trials at the time of the publication of this *Atlas*. Their place in history is still to be determined.

CONCLUSION

The centenary of Dr Alzheimer's description of the illness that bears his name is a timely moment to reflect on the history of AD and dementia. This chapter outlines human awareness of dementia going back several millennia and reminds us that there is much to be learned through the consideration of history. The last few decades have been filled with huge scientific discovery, and create the hope that the next will bear the fruit of therapy for the community afflicted by this disease.

REFERENCES

1. Schafer D. 'That senescence itself is an illness': a transitional medical concept of age and ageing in the eighteenth century. Med Hist, 2002; 46: 525–48.

2. Berchtold NC, Cotman CW. Evolution in the conceptualization of dementia and Alzheimer's disease: Greco-Roman period to the 1960s. Neurobiol Aging, 1998; 19: 173–89.

3. Halpert BP. Development of the term 'senility' as a medical diagnosis. Minn Med, 1983; 66: 421–4.

4. Boller F, Forbes MM. History of dementia and dementia in history: an overview. J Neurol Sci, 1998; 158: 125–33.

5. Beach TG. The history of Alzheimer's disease: three debates. J Hist Med Allied Sci, 1987; 42: 327–49.

6. Graeber MB, Mehraein P. Reanalysis of the first case of Alzheimer's disease. Eur Arch Psychiatry Clin Neurosci, 1999; 249 (Suppl 3): 10–13.

7. Berrios GE. Alzheimer's disease: A conceptual history. Int J Geriatr Psychiatry, 1990; 5 (6): 355–65.

8. Maurer K, Volk S, Gerbaldo H. Auguste D and Alzheimer's disease. Lancet, 1997; 349: 1546–9.

9. Amaducci LA, Rocca WA, Schoenberg BS. Origin of the distinction between Alzheimer's disease and senile dementia: how history can clarify nosology. Neurology, 1986; 36: 1497–9.

10. Graeber MB, Kosel S, Egensperger R et al. Rediscovery of the case described by Alois Alzheimer in 1911: historical, histological and molecular genetic analysis. Neurogenetics, 1997; 1: 73–80.

11. Holstein M. Alzheimer's disease and senile dementia, 1885–1920: An interpretive history of disease negotiation. J Aging Studies, 1997; 11(1): 1–13.

12. Katzman R. Alzheimer's disease. N Engl J Med, 1986; 314: 964–73.

13. Katzman R, Jackson JE. Alzheimer disease: basic and clinical advances. J Am Geriatr Soc, 1991; 39: 516–25.

14. Tomlinson BE, Blessed G, Roth M. Observations on the brains of non-demented old people. J Neurol Sci, 1968; 7: 331–56.

15. Tomlinson BE, Blessed G, Roth M. Observations on the brains of demented old people. J Neurol Sci, 1970; 11: 205–42.

16. Whitehouse PJ, Price DL, Struble RG. Alzheimer's disease and senile dementia: loss of neurons in the basal forebrain. Science, 1982; 215: 1237–39.

17. Heston LL, Mastri AR, Anderson VE, White J. Dementia of the Alzheimer type. Clinical genetics, natural history, and associated conditions. Arch Gen Psychiatry, 1981; 38: 1085–90.

18. Glenner GG, Wong CW. Alzheimer's disease and Down's syndrome: sharing of a unique cerebrovascular amyloid fibril protein. Biochem Biophys Res Commun, 1984; 122: 1131–5.

19. Kang J, Lemaire HG, Unterbeck A et al. The precursor of Alzheimer's disease amyloid A4 protein resembles a cell-surface receptor. Nature, 1987; 325: 733–6.

20. St George-Hyslop P, Haines J, Rogaev E et al. Genetic evidence for a novel familial Alzheimer's disease locus on chromosome 14. Nat Genet, 1992; 2: 330–4.

21. Levy-Lahad E, Wijsman EM, Nemens E et al. A familial Alzheimer's disease locus on chromosome 1. Science, 1995; 269: 970–3.

22. Tanzi RE, Bertram L. Twenty years of the Alzheimer's disease amyloid hypothesis: a genetic perspective. Cell, 2005; 120: 545–55.

23. Saunders AM, Strittmatter WJ, Schmechel D et al. Association of apolipoprotein E allele E4 with late-onset familial and sporadic Alzheimer's disease. Neurology, 1993; 43: 1467–72.

24. Corder EH, Saunders AM, Strittmatter WJ et al. Gene dose of apoliprotein E type 4 allele and the risk of Alzheimer's disease in late onset families. Science, 1993; 261: 921–3.

25. Foster NL, Wilhelmsen K, Sima AA et al. Frontotemporal dementia and parkinsonism linked to chromosome 17: a consensus conference. Ann Neurol 1997; 41: 706–15.

26. Hardy J, Allsop D. Amyloid deposition as the central event in the aetiology of Alzheimer's disease. Trends Pharmacol Sci, 1991; 12(10): 383–8.

27. Hardy JA, Higgins GA. Alzheimer's disease: the amyloid cascade hypothesis. Science, 1992; 256: 184–5.

28. Hsiao K, Chapman P, Nilsen S et al. Correlative memory deficits, Abeta elevation, and amyloid plaques in transgenic mice. Science, 1996; 274: 99–102.

29. Pereira C, Agostinho P, Moreira PI, Cardoso SM, Oliveira CR. Alzheimer's disease-associated neurotoxic mechanisms and neuroprotective strategies. Curr Drug Targets CNS Neurol Disord, 2005; 4: 383–403.

30. Scheltens P, Korf ES. Contribution of neuroimaging in the diagnosis of Alzheimer's disease and other dementias. Curr Opin Neurol, 2000; 13: 391–6.

31. Agdeppa ED, Kepe V, Liu J et al. Binding characteristics of radiofluorinated 6-dialkylamino-2-naphthylethylidene derivatives as positron emission tomography imaging probes for beta-amyloid plaques in Alzheimer's disease. J Neurosci, 2001; 21: RC189.

32. Nordberg A. PET imaging of amyloid in Alzheimer's disease. Lancet Neurol, 2004; 3: 519–27.

33. APA (American Psychiatric Association). Diagnostic and Statistical Manual of Mental Disorders, DSM-III-R edn. Washington, DC: American Psychiatric Association, 1987.

34. McKhann G, Drachman DA, Folstein M et al. Clinical diagnosis of Alzheimer's disease – Report of the NINCDS-

ADRDA Work Group under the auspices of Department of Health and Human Services Task Force on Alzheimer's disease. Neurology, 1984; 34: 939–44.

35. Khachaturian ZS. Diagnosis of Alzheimer's disease. Arch Neurol, 1985; 42: 1097–105.

36. Hyman BT, Trojanowski JQ. Consensus recommendations for the postmortem diagnosis of Alzheimer disease from the National Institute on Aging and the Reagan Institute Working Group on diagnostic criteria for the neuropathological assessment of Alzheimer disease [editorial]. J Neuropathol Exp Neurol, 1997; 56: 1095–7.

37. Folstein MF, Folstein S, McHugh PR. Mini-mental state: a practical method for grading the cognitive state of patients for the clinician. J Psychiatr Res, 1975; 12: 189–98.

38. Rosen WG, Mohs RC, Davis KL. A new rating scale for Alzheimer's disease. Am J Psychiatry, 1984; 141 (11): 1356–64.

39. Sheikh K, Smith DS, Meade TW et al. Repeatability and validity of a modified activities of daily living (ADL) index in studies of chronic disability. Int Rehabil Med, 1979; 1: 51–8.

40. Gelinas I, Gauthier L, McIntyre M, Gauthier S. Development of a functional measure for persons with Alzheimer's disease: The Disability Assessment for Dementia. Am J Occup Ther, 1999; 53: 471–81.

41. Cummings JL, Mega M, Gray K et al. The Neuropsychiatric Inventory (NPI). Neurology, 1994; 44: 2308–14.

42. Reisberg B, Borenstein J, Salob SP. Behavioral symptoms in Alzheimer's disease: phenomenology and treatment. J Clin Psychiatry, 1987; 48(Suppl), 9–15.

43. Knopman DS, Knapp MJ, Gracon SI, Davis CS. The Clinician Interview-Based Impression (CIBI): a clinician's global change rating scale in Alzheimer's disease. Neurology, 1994; 44: 2315–21.

44. Hughes CP, Berg L, Danzinger WL. A new clinical scale for the staging of dementia. Bri J Psychiatry, 1982; 140: 566–72.

45. Peters BH, Levin HS. Effects of physotigmine and lecithin on memory in Alzheimer disease. Ann Neurol, 1979; 6(3): 219–21.

46. Bliss TV, Collingridge GL. A synaptic model of memory: long-term potentiation in the hippocampus. Nature, 1993; 361: 31–9.

47. Sucher NJ, Awobuluyi M, Choi YB, Lipton SA. NMDA receptors: from genes to channels. Trends Pharmacol Sci, 1996; 17: 348–55.

48. Areosa Sastre A, Sherriff F, McShane R. Memantine for Dementia. The Cochrane Database of Systematic Reviews. 25-5-2005.

CHAPTER 2

Epidemiology of Alzheimer's disease and dementia
Ging-Yuek Robin Hsiung

INTRODUCTION

Epidemiology is the study of the occurrence of disease in the human population. The two main purposes of epidemiologic studies are (1) to describe the frequency and distribution of disease, and (2) to identify risk factors responsible for disease. The first function assists our planning for health care and determines health priorities, while the second helps to guide treatment and ultimately lead to preventive strategies for disease. The knowledge on the epidemiology of Alzheimer's disease (AD) and dementia has advanced considerably in the past decade. In this chapter, the epidemiology of AD and dementia will be described with the liberal use of graphs. Non-modifiable risk factors of AD and dementia, namely age, gender, education, and genetic factors, will also be discussed here. Modifiable risk factors such as blood pressure, cholesterol level, smoking, and others will be examined in detail in a subsequent chapter on prevention of AD (Chapter 6).

DESCRIPTIVE EPIDEMIOLOGY

When describing the occurrence of disease, two concepts are often used. Prevalence refers to the proportion of a population affected by a disease at a specific point in time, while incidence describes the number of new cases of a disease that occur in a population at risk during a given time period (i.e. over one year), and estimates the risk of an individual of becoming ill.[1] Prevalence (P) is affect by both the incidence (I) and the duration (D) of a disease.

$$P = I \times D$$

For diseases that lead to death shortly after diagnosis (e.g. Creutzfeldt–Jakob disease), the prevalence and incidence are essentially the same. By contrast, for diseases with a long survival after diagnosis (e.g. multiple sclerosis), the prevalence is a much larger number than incidence, reflecting the prolonged duration of illness. While prevalence estimates the risk of an individual getting the disease at a certain point in time in a defined population and provides a public health perspective on disease burden, incidence reflects the risk of an individual becoming sick with the disease at a given period of time. Incidence rate may be used to quantify the impact of a treatment or prevention strategy, and is a convenient way to measure risk factors of a disease.

Prevalence of dementia around the world

Dementia has become one of the leading public health concerns as our population ages. In North America, 6–10% of persons aged 65 or older suffer from some form of dementia.[2–4] There have been many studies conducted on the prevalence of dementia throughout the world, although most have been concentrated in the developed countries.[3–22] However, with the continuous decline in mortality and fertility rates in the developing countries, aging of the population has now become a worldwide phenomenon and is no longer limited to the developed Western societies.[7] In fact, the aging process of a population is currently most prominent in the developing countries. In a report by Ferri et al, it is estimated that 24.3 million people in the world were suffering from dementia in 2001, with an estimated 4.6 million new cases every year.[5] This is equivalent to one new case every 7 seconds. The number of people affected by dementia is projected to double approximately every 20 years to 42.3 million in 2020, and to 81.1 million by 2040.[5]

Figure 2.1 illustrates the effect of age on the prevalence of dementia across six world regions. Although the estimates vary widely among different regions, the exponential growth pattern with increasing age is consistent throughout, with the prevalence doubling approximately every 5 years of increase in age. The percentage prevalence estimates within each age group are comparable in Europe, America, Middle East, and North Africa, as well as Western Pacific, while lower estimates are seen in parts of South Asia and Africa, where overall life expectancy is lower. Figure 2.2(a) shows a more detailed breakdown of the percentage prevalence by 5-year age group in each of the WHO world regions, which are based on geography. For reference, a map of these regions is shown in Figure 2.2(b).

While the prevalence of dementia was comparably high in China, Western Europe, and North America in 2001 (Figure 2.3), it will be overshadowed by the growth in prevalence in the developing countries, especially in China and South East Asia, within the next 40 years. Compared to other regions, Africa has the lowest increase in prevalence, which is likely a reflection of the higher child and adult mortality within this region, with a considerable proportion of the population not reaching the mean age of onset of dementia.

Prevalence of Alzheimer's disease and subtypes of dementia

As for the prevalence of dementia, the prevalence of AD in different countries shows a similar exponential increase with increasing age.[7] While AD is the most common cause of dementia, there are other neurodegenerative and medical causes of dementia. The proportions of the subtypes vary by age of onset and geographic region, as well as by method of ascertainment. In a cohort of patients referred to specialized dementia clinics across Canada, AD as the solo etiology represented close to half of all the patients diagnosed with dementia across all ages (Figure 2.4a).[23] However, frontotemporal dementia was significantly more frequent in the younger age group (<70 years old) compared to the older age group (12.1% vs 2%), while mixed vascular dementia with AD was significantly more common in the older age group (23% vs 9%) (Figure 2.4b).

In a study of early onset dementia patients (age <65 years) seen in a Veterans Affairs Medical Center in the US, it was noted that vascular dementia was the most frequent diagnosis (29%), followed by traumatic brain injury (24%) and early onset AD (17%).[24] However, this study utilized a specialized sample from the veteran population (97% male, who might have been exposed to different sets of risk factors); therefore, the findings may not be generalizable to other populations (Figure 2.5). Nevertheless, it highlights the variation in the patterns observed in different age groups and different populations.

In a post-mortem study of dementia causes, solo AD pathology was found in slightly less than 50% of cases (Figure 2.6a).[25] There is a significant trend, with lower frequency of co-existing Lewy body dementia and frontotemporal dementia with increasing age, while a higher frequency of vascular dementia (pure or mixed) was observed with older age (Figure 2.6b).

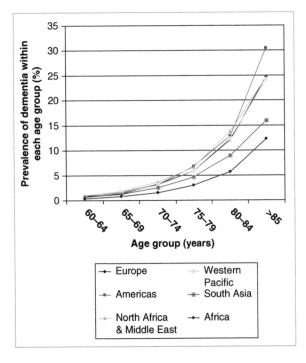

Figure 2.1 Prevalence of dementia in 6 WHO world regions (based on data extracted from Ferri et al. Global prevalence of dementia: a Delphi consensus study. Lancet 2005; 366: 211–17).[5]

(a)

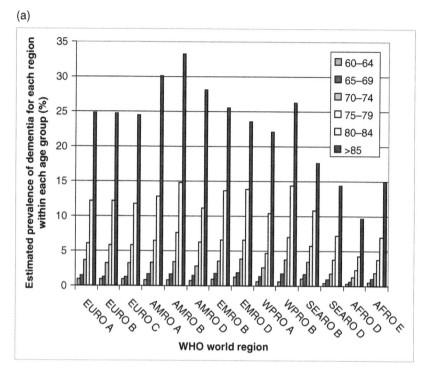

Figure 2.2 (a) Estimated prevalence of dementia for each WHO world region by age group (%). The WHO world regions are defined by geography (AMRO [the Americas], EURO [Europe], EMRO [North Africa and the Middle East], AFRO [Africa], SEARO [South Asia], and WPRO [Western Pacific], and patterns of child and adult mortality, from A (lowest) to E (highest). (Data extracted from Ferri et al. Global prevalence of dementia: a Delphi consensus study. Lancet 2005; 366: 2112–17).[5]

Continued...

Comparisons by ethnicity and world region also show variations with the proportion of AD, vascular dementia, and other dementias (Figure 2.7). AD represents nearly three-quarters of all dementias in North America, especially in the African-American population, while it is lower at about 50% in Asia and Asian-Americans.[4,7,26] By contrast, vascular dementia is more common in Asia and Asian-Americans.

In countries of the Far East such as Japan, Korea, and China, vascular dementia was reportedly more common than AD in studies from the 1980s, while recent data show an increase in prevalence in AD with a relative decline in vascular dementia (Figure 2.8).[11,15,18,19,21,27–31] The change in disease pattern in these countries may be explained by a model of transition from a low incidence–high mortality society, to a high incidence–high mortality society, to a low incidence–low mortality society, as hypothesized by Suh and Shah.[32] The overall increase in prevalence reflects the aging of a population. As more people reach the age at risk for AD, there is a proportionate rise in incidence. Improvement in socio-eonomic conditions and advances in medical treatment also prolong the survival after onset of disease, further contributing to the increase in prevalence of AD. By contrast, the observed decrease in prevalence of vascular dementia is hypothesized to be due to a lower incidence with improved preventive measures as health awareness in the society progressed.

Incidence of dementia and Alzheimer's disease

While a large number of prevalence studies on dementia have been done, especially in the developed world, incidence studies are less frequent, probably because they are much more costly to conduct. Based on the available studies, it has been shown consistently that the incidence of dementia rises sharply with age from about 2–5 per 1000 person-years at age 60, to 40–110 per 1000 person-years at age 85 years (Figure 2.9).[6,33–40] The variation in the findings among different parts of the world, and sometimes even within a country, may be due to a number of reasons. There are methodologic differences, such as the different criteria used for diagnosing dementia, and the different data-collection and sampling methods. It may also reflect the different age structure of each population, or the different rate of exposure to environmental and genetic risk factors for dementia in different populations. Of interest is that, in several studies, there was a decline in incidence after age 90.[33,35,40] A similar pattern was also observed with the incidence rate studies of AD. The number rose exponentially with increasing

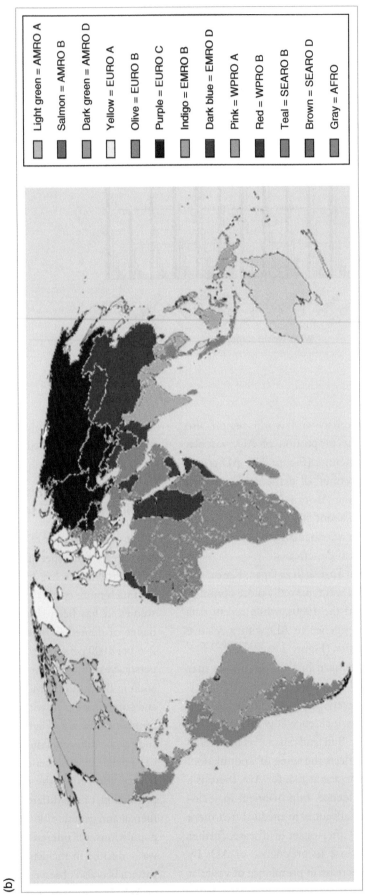

(b)

Light green = AMRO A
Salmon = AMRO B
Dark green = AMRO D
Yellow = EURO A
Olive = EURO B
Purple = EURO C
Indigo = EMRO B
Dark blue = EMRO D
Pink = WPRO A
Red = WPRO B
Teal = SEARO B
Brown = SEARO D
Gray = AFRO

Figure 2.2 Continued...(b) Map of the WHO world regions represented in Figure 2.2(a).

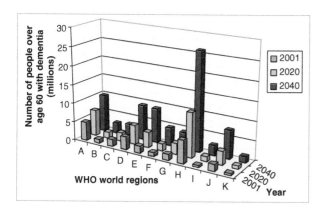

Figure 2.3 Projected prevalence of dementia in the years 2020 and 2040, as compared to 2001, in the main regions of the world. A = Western Europe (EURO A), B = Eastern Europe with low adult mortality (EURO B), C = Eastern Europe with high adult mortality (EURO C), D = North America (AMRO A), E = Latin America (AMRO B/D), F = North Africa and Eastern Mediterranean (EMRO B/D), G = developed Western Pacific (WPRO A), H = China and developing Western Pacific (WPRO B), I = Indonesia, Thailand, and Sri Lanka (SEARO B), J = India and South Asia (SEARO D), K = Africa (AFRO D/E). (Data extracted from Ferri et al. Global prevalence of dementia: a Delphi consensus study. Lancet 2005; 366: 2112–17).[5]

age across all studies, but a few exhibited a decline after 90 years of age (Figure 2.10).[6,16,36,39–42] One source of discrepancy is the rather small numbers in this age group, and a detailed breakdown of this age category is not available in most studies. However, if this finding is indeed true, it would be consistent with the hypothesis that genetic factors predispose a person to develop AD, while other factors modulate the age of onset of clinical dementia. One might hypothesize that those who survive through to this old age and remain cognitively intact have escaped the inheritance of the predisposing genetic risk factors. Some research studies are currently concentrating on this 'oldest old' population in an attempt to identify the 'protective factors' against AD and dementia.[43–46]

Survival after diagnosis of dementia and Alzheimer's disease

Since prevalence is determined by incidence and duration of illness, life expectancy following the diagnosis of chronic diseases such as dementia and AD provides important information for health planners, families, and patients, as well as caregivers. Earlier estimates of survival range widely from 1.8 to over 16 years.[47] Some argued that these studies might have underestimated the

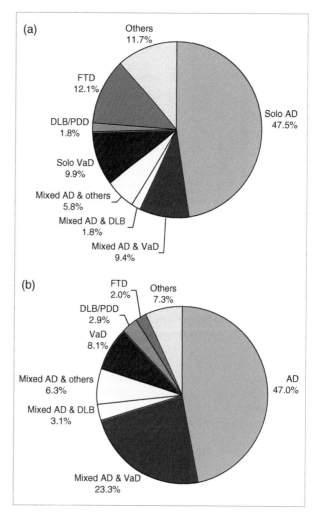

Figure 2.4 (a) Causes of dementia in patients <70 years old. (b) Causes of dementia in patients 70 years or older. (Data extracted from Feldman et al. AD, Alzheimer Disease; DLB, Dementia with Lewy Body; FTD, Frontotemporal Dementia; PDD, Parkinson Disease with Dementia; VaD, Vascular Dementia. A Canadian cohort study of cognitive impairment and related dementias (ACCORD): study methods and baseline results. Neuroepidemiology 2003; 22: 265–74).[23]

severity of dementia as these studies were based on follow-up of prevalent cases; hence, persons who died shortly following a diagnosis were often excluded from the analysis. This resulting bias is termed 'length bias' as described by Wolfson et al.[48] In their study using data from the Canadian Study of Health and Aging (mean age at sampling was 83.8 years), the unadjusted median survival was 6.6 years (95% CI 6.2–7.1), whereas the survival after adjustment of length bias was 3.3 years

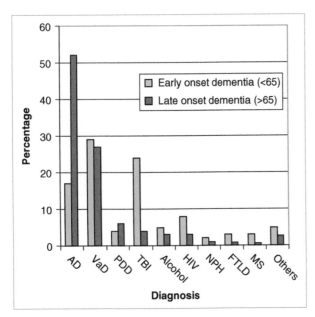

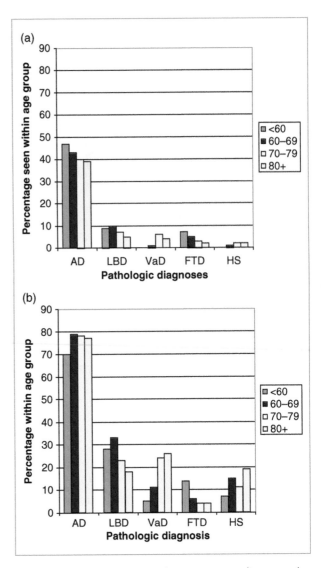

Figure 2.5 Proportions of dementia etiologies in early onset vs late onset from a Veteran's Affair Medical Center. AD = Alzheimer's disease, VaD = vascular dementia, PDD = Parkinsonian disorders with dementia (including Parkinson's disease, Lewy body disease, multiple systems atrophy, corticobasal degeneration, and progressive supranuclear palsy), TBI = traumatic brain injury, NPH = normal pressure hydrocephalus, FTLD = frontotemporal lobar degeneration, and MS = multiple sclerosis. (Modified with permission from McMurtray et al. Early-onset dementia: frequency and causes compared to late-onset dementia. Dement Geriatr Cogn Disord 2006; 21: 59–64.[24] Copyright © 2006).

Figure 2.6 (a) Frequency of post-mortem diagnoses by age at onset with pure pathologic findings. (b) Frequency of post-mortem diagnoses by age at onset allowing for mixed pathologic findings. AD = Alzheimer's disease, LBD = Lewy body dementia, VaD = vascular dementia, FTD = frontotemporal dementia, and HS = hippocampal sclerosis. (Data extracted from Barker et al. Relative frequencies of Alzheimer disease, Lewy body, vascular and frontotemporal dementia, and hippocampal sclerosis in the State of Florida Brain Bank. Alzheimer Dis Assoc Disord 2002; 16: 203–12).

(95% CI 2.7–4.0). In a study from the Baltimore Longitudinal Study of Aging, it was found that the median survival time following a diagnosis of AD depends strongly on the patient's age at diagnosis (Figure 2.11).[49] The median survival time was 8.3 years for people diagnosed at age 65 or younger, 6.0 years for age 65 to 75, 5.0 years for age 75 through 84, and 3.5 years for age 85 or older.

The mortality of AD patients is further associated with the rate of cognitive decline. In a study comparing the risk of death by the rate of cognitive decline divided in quartiles and using the slowest decline as the reference, those in quartile 2 had a 3-fold increased risk of death, quartile 3 had a 5-fold increase, and quartile 4 (fastest rate of cognitive decline) had a greater than 8-fold increased risk (Figure 2.12).[50] The survival rate may increase as dementia care improves and newer therapies become available.

Effect of delaying onset of Alzheimer's disease

As mentioned above, the alarmingly high prevalence of dementia and AD in our aging population emphasizes the importance for public health planning in the near future. The potential impact of an intervention that may delay the onset of AD was estimated in a study by

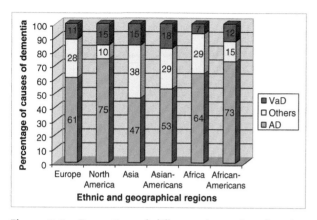

Figure 2.7 Proportion of different dementing disorders in different continents and ethnicity. (Data extracted from Fratiglioni et al. Worldwide prevalence and incidence of dementia. Drugs Aging 1999; 15: 365–75).[7]

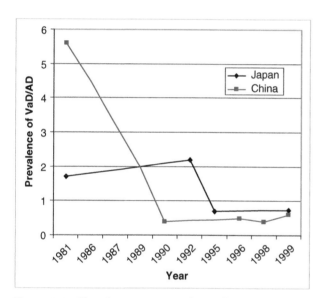

Figure 2.8 The change in ratio of prevalence of vascular dementia vs Alzheimer's disease in Japan and China over the last two decades.[11,15,18,19,27–30]

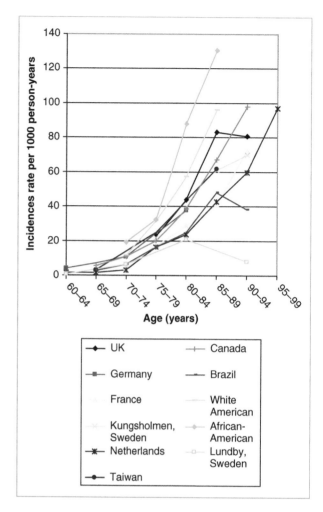

Figure 2.9 Age-specific incidence rates of dementia per 1000 person-years. (Data derived from selected studies).[6,33–40]

professionals to care for these patients. It is also imperative to set research priorities and allocation of resources.

RISK FACTORS OF ALZHEIMER'S DISEASE

While descriptive epidemiology helps to assess the impact of disease burden in a population, analytic epidemiologic studies are important for identification of disease risk factors. In general, risk factors may be divided into non-modifiable and modifiable ones. Those that are modifiable are obvious targets for preventive treatment and will be discussed in another chapter, while non-modifiable ones are still important in understanding the pathogenesis of the disease, these include age, sex, level of education, family history, and genetic factors.

Brookmeyer et al[51] (Figure 2.13). According to their estimates, if the onset of AD can be delayed by 5 years, the number of affected people in the USA will decrease by almost 50% by the middle of the century. Even with a modest delay by one year, the prevalence will decrease by close to one million.

As the number of older people in a population increases, it is important to prepare for the increasing need for appropriate housing and other services, and for health

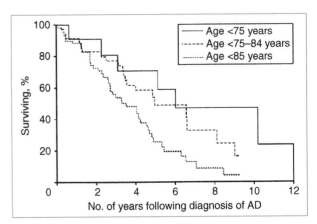

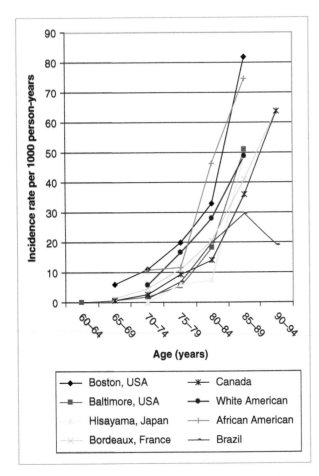

Figure 2.11 Survival after diagnosis of AD by age of onset. (Reprinted from Brookmeyer et al. Survival following a diagnosis of Alzheimer disease. Arch Neurol 2002; 59: 1764–7.[49] Copyright © 2002, American Medical Association. All rights reserved).

Figure 2.10 Age-specific incidence of Alzheimer's disease per 1000 person-years in selected studies.[6,16,36,39–42]

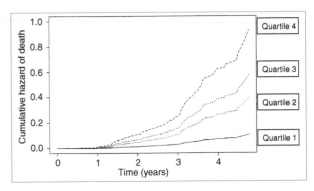

Figure 2.12 Cumulative hazard of death as a function of time, stratified by quartiles according to rate of cognitive decline. Quartile 1, with the least decline, is represented by a solid line, quartile 2 by a dotted line, quartile 3 by a short-dashed line, quartile 4, the subgroup with the most rapid decline, with a long-dashed line. (Reprinted from Hui et al. Rate of cognitive decline and mortality in Alzheimer's disease. Neurology 2003; 61: 1356–61).[50]

Age

As demonstrated in the incidence and prevalence studies of AD (Figures 2.9 and 2.10), age is the most consistent risk factor demonstrated across all studies.[4,6,7,39,52,53] This is perhaps a reflection of the pathologic process of amyloid plaque formation over time. The longer a person lives, the longer the time there is for plaque accumulation, and the more likely that clinical dementia will be expressed. In addition, the aging brain is exposed to a lifetime of changes, and small insults such as oxidative stress, trauma, damaged molecules, inflammation, and white matter disease from small vessel ischemia may slowly accumulate over the years to eventually become symptomatic after a threshold is reached. Therefore, this cumulative damage to the brain is much more likely to manifest cognitive deficits in an older individual.

Gender

In most studies, women were found to be at greater risk for AD, while men appeared to be at a somewhat higher risk for vascular dementia.[4,7,37,39,40,54–57] The effect of gender and age on incidence of AD is shown in Figure 2.14.[58] This finding is robust even after adjustment for differences in survival and level of education. However, whether the effect is due to genetic or hormonal differences between males and females or a surrogate marker of other unmeasured socioeconomic factors is still under investigation. Another argument is

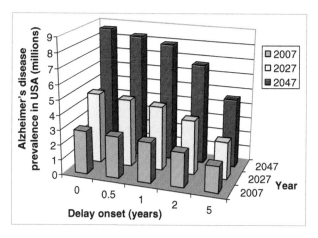

Figure 2.13 Potential effect on prevalence by interventions to delay the onset of Alzheimer's disease. (Based on data extracted from Brookmeyer et al. Projections of Alzheimer's disease in the United States and the public health impact of delaying disease onset. Am J Public Health 1998; 88: 1337–42).[51]

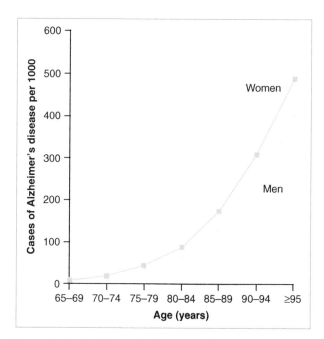

Figure 2.14 Incidence of Alzheimer's disease as a function of age in men and women. (Reprinted with permission from Nussbaum RL, Ellis CE. Alzheimer's disease and Parkinson's disease. N Engl J Med 2003; 348: 1356–64).[58]

that the higher prevalence of cerebrovascular disease in men may lead to overdiagnosis of vascular dementia, and consequently an artificial increase in the proportion of women diagnosed with AD.

Level of education

A number of studies have found that a low educational level increases the risk for dementia and AD.[19,59–63] Data

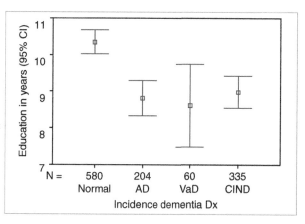

Figure 2.15 Effect of education on the incidence of cognitively impaired not demented (CIND), Alzheimer's disease (AD), and vascular dementia (VaD) from the Canadian Study of Health and Aging. (Reproduced with permission from Hsiung et al. Apolipoprotein E epsilon4 genotype as a risk factor for cognitive decline and dementia: data from the Canadian Study of Health and Aging. CMAJ 2004; 171: 863–7).[63] Copyright © 2004 Massachusetts Medical Society. All rights reserved.

from the Canadian Study on Health and Aging show that a lower level of education is associated with a higher risk of AD and vascular dementia, as well as with the state of cognitively impaired not demented (CIND)[63] (Figure 2.15). However, years of education, occupation, and other markers of socioeconomic status have also been associated with other chronic diseases of older people; therefore, it is possible that this association is not

Table 2.1 Relative risk of AD for individuals with a positive family history vs those who do not

Number of first-degree relatives affected	Age of onset (years)	Relative risk	95% CI
1	60–69	5.3	2.8–10
1	70–79	2.3	1.4–4.6
1	80 and over	2.6	1.3–5.2
1	Overall	3.5	2.6–4.6
2 or more	Overall	7.5	3.3–8.7

Data extracted from van Duijn et al. Familial aggregation of Alzheimer's disease and related disorders: a collaborative re-analysis of case-control studies. EURODEM Risk Factors Research Group. Int J Epidemiol 1991; 20 (Suppl 2): S13–20.[68]

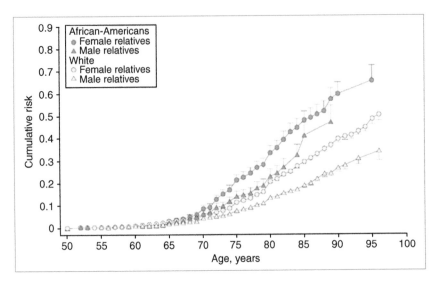

Figure 2.16 Cumulative risk of dementia in first-degree biological relatives of Alzheimer's disease probands, stratified by relatives' sex and ethnicity. (Reprinted with permission from Green et al. Risk of dementia among white and African American relatives of patients with Alzheimer disease. JAMA 2002; 287: 329–36.[69] Copyright © 2002, American Medical Association. All rights reserved).

specific for AD or dementia. Others have argued that the less educated may be worse at taking cognitive tests. One study reported that linguistic ability in early adult life predicted both level of cognitive function before death and AD pathology.[64] Another study found that lower childhood mental ability scores were associated with a higher risk of late-onset dementia.[65] These findings led to the hypothesis that lifetime cognitive experience may influence the number of neurons and synapses that survive into adult life (cognitive reserve hypothesis) – the greater the number of synapses formed between neurons, the longer the time needed for the synapses to degenerate, and the later the onset of dementia.[66,67]

Family history and ethnicity

Many studies have shown that family history is a risk factor for AD, especially for occurrence in a first-degree relative (parent or sibling). Data from the EURODEM case-control studies show that the overall risk of AD with a single first-degree relative is 3.5 (95% CI 2.6–4.6).[68] The change in relative risk by age of onset is shown in Table 2.1. The risk is greatest in those with age of onset between 60 and 69, but is still significant in older age groups. Individuals with two or more first-degree relatives affected have an even higher risk (RR 7.5, 95% CI 3.3–8.7).[68]

In another study that examined the lifetime dementia risk among relatives of white and African-American probands diagnosed with probable or definite AD, it was found that first-degree relatives of African-Americans

with AD have a higher cumulative risk of dementia than those of whites.[69] The cumulative risks in relatives of Alzheimer patients compared to that of spouses (controls) in African-Americans and whites are shown in Figure 2.16.

Genetic factors

Currently, four genes have been found to be definitely associated with AD. The properties of these four genes are summarized in Table 2.2. Mutations in the amyloid precursor protein (APP), presenilin 1 (PS1), and presenilin 2 (PS2) are known to cause early onset Alzheimer disease, with PS1 mutations being the most frequent.[70] Molecular studies of these three mutations are all associated with an increased production of the Aβ42 amyloid peptide, and provide support for the amyloid cascade hypothesis of AD pathogenesis. By contrast, apolipo-protein E (ApoE) is a susceptibility risk factor, as it is neither necessary nor sufficient to cause AD. It is a molecular chaperone which is involved in cholesterol trafficking in the brain.[71] It exists in three common polymorphisms: ε2, ε3, and ε4. The effect of ε4 on the risk of AD is strongest in homozygous carriers with a large effect from age 40 to 80, with a peak around age 60–65 (Figure 2.17a). There is also an interaction effect with sex (Figure 2.17b); that is, female ε4 carriers are at a higher risk of developing AD than male ε4 carriers, especially from age 55 to 85. The ε4 genotype also increases risk of conversion from cognitive impairment to dementia, but the low sensitivity and specificity

36

Table 2.2 Genes associated with Alzheimer's disease

Chromosome	Gene	Penetrance of mutated gene	Frequency in familial AD with known mutations	Mutation	Pathology
21q21	APP	High penetrance	About 18% of familial early onset AD	Missense mutations around Aβ portion of APP	Increases $A\beta_{42}$ production during APP processing
14q24.3	PS1	High penetrance	Represent up to 78% of familial early onset AD	Mostly missense mutations	Promotes cleavage at γ-secretase site and increase Aβ production and accumulation
1q31.42	PS2	Incomplete penetrance	Rare, ~4%	Missense mutations	Promotes cleavage at β-secretase site leading to increased Aβ production and accumulation

Chromosome	Gene	Susceptiblity factor	Allele frequency in population	Mutation	Pathology
19q13.2	APOE	Risk factor, but neither necessary nor sufficient to cause AD	ε2 ~10% ε3 ~75% ε4 ~15%	ε4 genotype, heterozygous increases odds by ~3, and homozygous by ~9	Acts as a molecular chaperone to promote Aβ accumulation and senile plaque formation

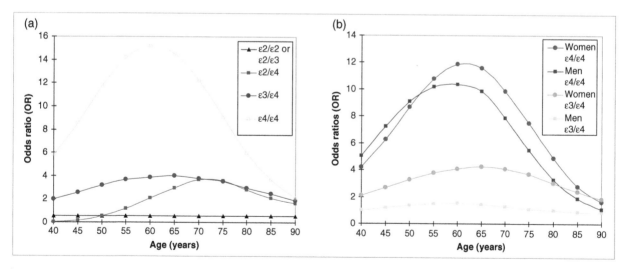

Figure 2.17 (a) Relative odds of Alzheimer's disease based on APOE genotypes ε2, ε3/ε4 and ε4/ε4 by age, compared to ε3/ε3 carriers as reference OR = 1. (b) Relative odds of Alzheimer's disease based on APOE genotypes ε3/ε4 and ε4/ε4, age, and sex, compared to ε3/ε3 as reference OR = 1. (Reproduced with permission from Farrer et al. Effects of age, sex, and ethnicity on the association between apolipoprotein E genotype and Alzheimer disease. A meta-analysis. APOE and Alzheimer Disease Meta Analysis Consortium. JAMA 1997; 278: 1349–56.[72] Copyright © 1997, American Medical Association. All rights reserved).

preclude its use as a diagnostic tool for AD, or for screening in the general population.[63,73] Nevertheless, it is an important genetic risk factor and accounts for 7–17% of the variance in age of onset of AD, and may contribute up to 50% of the genetic risks of AD in the US.[74-78] There are likely several other genes that confer risk to AD, and linkage analyses on families with AD have revealed significant LOD scores on chromosomes 9, 10, 12, and 19.[74,75,79-83] To date, many candidate genes for AD have been proposed and examined, but none other than the four mentioned have been consistently replicated so far.[70,71]

SUMMARY

In conclusion, epidemiologic studies have demonstrated that AD is a significant burden to our current and future health care system, not only in the developed countries, but even more so in the developing countries. Identifying the risk factors for AD will clearly help control or prevent this epidemic. Further research on the prevention and treatment of this devastating and costly disease should be a priority.

REFERENCES

1. Rothman K, Greenland S. Modern Epidemiology. Philadelphia: Lippincott-Raven, 1998.

2. Kukull WA, Ganguli M. Epidemiology of dementia: concepts and overview. Neurol Clin 2000; 18: 923–50.

3. CSHA. Canadian study of health and aging: study methods and prevalence of dementia. CMAJ 1994; 150: 899–913.

4. Hendrie HC. Epidemiology of dementia and Alzheimer's disease. Am J Geriatr Psychiatry 1998; 6: S3–18.

5. Ferri CP, Prince M, Brayne C et al. Global prevalence of dementia: a Delphi consensus study. Lancet 2005; 366: 2112–17.

6. Fitzpatrick AL, Kuller LH, Ives DG et al. Incidence and prevalence of dementia in the Cardiovascular Health Study. J Am Geriatr Soc 2004; 52: 195–204.

7. Fratiglioni L, De Ronchi D, Aguero-Torres H. Worldwide prevalence and incidence of dementia. Drugs Aging 1999; 15: 365–75.

8. Hamad AI, Ibrahim MA, Sulaiti EM. Dementia in Qatar. Saudi Med J 2004; 25: 79–82.

9. Jellinger K. Prevalence of Alzheimer's disease in very elderly people: a prospective neuropathological study. Neurology 2002; 58: 671–2; author reply 671–2.

10. Lin RT, Lai CL, Tai CT et al. Prevalence and subtypes of dementia in southern Taiwan: impact of age, sex, education, and urbanization. J Neurol Sci 1998; 160: 67–75.

11. Liu CK, Lin RT, Chen YF et al. Prevalence of dementia in an urban area in Taiwan. J Formos Med Assoc 1996; 95: 7628.

12. Liu HC, Fuh JL, Wang SJ et al. Prevalence and subtypes of dementia in a rural Chinese population. Alzheimer Dis Assoc Disord 1998; 12: 127–34.

13. Lobo A, Launer LJ, Fratiglioni L et al. Prevalence of dementia and major subtypes in Europe: a collaborative study of population-based cohorts. Neurologic Diseases in the Elderly Research Group. Neurology 2000; 54: S4–9.

14. Rice DP, Fillit HM, Max W et al. Prevalence, costs, and treatment of Alzheimer's disease and related dementia: a managed care perspective. Am J Manag Care 2001; 7: 809–18.

15. Ogura C, Nakamoto H, Uema T et al. Prevalence of senile dementia in Okinawa, Japan. COSEPO Group. Study Group of Epidemiology for Psychiatry in Okinawa. Int J Epidemiol 1995; 24: 373–80.

16. Sayetta RB. Rates of senile dementia, Alzheimer's type, in the Baltimore Longitudinal Study. J Chronic Dis 1986; 39: 271–86.

17. Shiba M, Shimogaito J, Kose A et al. Prevalence of dementia in the rural village of Hanazono-mura, Japan. Neuroepidemiology 1999; 18: 32–6.

18. Ueda K, Kawano H, Hasuo Y, Fujishima M. Prevalence and etiology of dementia in a Japanese community. Stroke 1992; 23: 798–803.

19. Zhang MY, Katzman R, Salmon D et al. The prevalence of dementia and Alzheimer's disease in Shanghai, China: impact of age, gender, and education. Ann Neurol 1990; 27: 428–37.

20. Yamada T, Kadekaru H, Matsumoto S et al. Prevalence of dementia in the older Japanese-Brazilian population. Psychiatry Clin Neurosci 2002; 56: 71–5.

21. Woo JI, Lee JH, Yoo KY et al. Prevalence estimation of dementia in a rural area of Korea. J Am Geriatr Soc 1998; 46: 983–7.

22. Henderson S. Epidemiology of dementia. Ann Med Interne (Paris) 1998; 149: 181–6.

23. Feldman H, Levy AR, Hsiung GY et al. A Canadian cohort study of cognitive impairment and related dementias (ACCORD): study methods and baseline results. Neuroepidemiology 2003; 22: 265–74.

24. McMurtray A, Clark DG, Christine D, Mendez MF. Early-onset dementia: frequency and causes compared to late-onset dementia. Dement Geriatr Cogn Disord 2006; 21: 59–64.

25. Barker WW, Luis CA, Kashuba A et al. Relative frequencies of Alzheimer disease, Lewy body, vascular and frontotemporal dementia, and hippocampal sclerosis in

the State of Florida Brain Bank. Alzheimer Dis Assoc Disord 2002; 16: 203–12.

26. White L, Petrovitch H, Ross GW et al. Prevalence of dementia in older Japanese-American men in Hawaii: The Honolulu-Asia Aging Study. JAMA 1996; 276: 955–60.

27. Hasegawa K. The clinical issues of age-related dementia. Tohoku J Exp Med 1990; 161(Suppl): 29–38.

28. Kuang PG. [A survey on senile mental disturbances in Wuhan City in 1981.] Zhonghua Liu Xing Bing Xue Za Zhi 1984; 5: 95–9.

29. Li G, Shen YC, Chen CH et al. An epidemiological survey of age-related dementia in an urban area of Beijing. Acta Psychiatr Scand 1989; 79: 557–63.

30. Yamada M, Sasaki H, Mimori Y et al. Prevalence and risks of dementia in the Japanese population: RERF's adult health study Hiroshima subjects. Radiation Effects Research Foundation. J Am Geriatr Soc 1999; 47: 189–95.

31. Park J, Ko HJ, Park YN, Jung CH. Dementia among the elderly in a rural Korean community. Br J Psychiatry 1994; 164: 796–801.

32. Suh GH, Shah A. A review of the epidemiological transition in dementia – cross-national comparisons of the indices related to Alzheimer's disease and vascular dementia. Acta Psychiatr Scand 2001; 104: 4–11.

33. Hagnell O, Lanke J, Rorsman B, Ojesjo L. Does the incidence of age psychosis decrease? A prospective, longitudinal study of a complete population investigated during the 25-year period 1947–1972: the Lundby study. Neuropsychobiology 1981; 7: 201–11.

34. Bickel H, Cooper B. Incidence and relative risk of dementia in an urban elderly population: findings of a prospective field study. Psychol Med 1994; 24: 179–92.

35. Boothby H, Blizard R, Livingston G, Mann AH. The Gospel Oak Study stage III: the incidence of dementia. Psychol Med 1994; 24: 89–95.

36. Letenneur L, Commenges D, Dartigues JF, Barberger-Gateau P. Incidence of dementia and Alzheimer's disease in elderly community residents of south-western France. Int J Epidemiol 1994; 23: 1256–61.

37. Fratiglioni L, Viitanen M, von Strauss E et al. Very old women at highest risk of dementia and Alzheimer's disease: incidence data from the Kungsholmen Project, Stockholm. Neurology 1997; 48: 132–8.

38. Liu CK, Lai CL, Tai CT et al. Incidence and subtypes of dementia in southern Taiwan: impact of socio-demographic factors. Neurology 1998; 50: 1572–9.

39. CSHA. The incidence of dementia in Canada. The Canadian Study of Health and Aging Working Group. Neurology 2000; 55: 66–73.

40. Nitrini R, Caramelli P, Herrera E Jr et al. Incidence of dementia in a community-dwelling Brazilian population. Alzheimer Dis Assoc Disord 2004; 18: 24–16.

41. Yoshitake T, Kiyohara Y, Kato I et al. Incidence and risk factors of vascular dementia and Alzheimer's disease in a defined elderly Japanese population: the Hisayama Study. Neurology 1995; 45: 1161–8.

42. Hebert LE, Scherr PA, Beckett LA et al. Age-specific incidence of Alzheimer's disease in a community population. JAMA 1995; 273: 1354–9.

43. Payami H, Grimslid H, Oken B et al. A prospective study of cognitive health in the elderly (Oregon Brain Aging Study): effects of family history and apolipoprotein E genotype. Am J Hum Genet 1997; 60: 948–56.

44. Gonzales McNeal M, Zareparsi S, Camicioli R et al. Predictors of healthy brain aging. J Gerontol A Biol Sci Med Sci 2001; 56: B294–301.

45. Johansson B, Hofer SM, Allaire JC et al. Change in cognitive capabilities in the oldest old: the effects of proximity to death in genetically related individuals over a 6-year period. Psychol Aging 2004; 19: 145–56.

46. Lautenschlager NT, Cupples LA, Rao VS et al. Risk of dementia among relatives of Alzheimer's disease patients in the MIRAGE study: what is in store for the oldest old? Neurology 1996; 46: 641–50.

47. Walsh JS, Welch HG, Larson EB. Survival of outpatients with Alzheimer-type dementia. Ann Intern Med 1990; 113: 429–34.

48. Wolfson C, Wolfson DB, Asgharian M et al. A reevaluation of the duration of survival after the onset of dementia. N Engl J Med 2001; 344: 1111–16.

49. Brookmeyer R, Corrada MM, Curriero FC, Kawas C. Survival following a diagnosis of Alzheimer disease. Arch Neurol 2002; 59: 1764–7.

50. Hui JS, Wilson RS, Bennett DA et al. Rate of cognitive decline and mortality in Alzheimer's disease. Neurology 2003; 61: 1356–61.

51. Brookmeyer R, Gray S, Kawas C. Projections of Alzheimer's disease in the United States and the public health impact of delaying disease onset. Am J Public Health 1998; 88: 1337–42.

52. Ott A, Breteler MM, van Harskamp F, Stijnen T, Hofman A. Incidence and risk of dementia. The Rotterdam Study. Am J Epidemiol 1998; 147: 574–80.

53. Fratiglioni L, Launer LJ, Andersen K et al. Incidence of dementia and major subtypes in Europe: a collaborative study of population-based cohorts. Neurologic Diseases in the Elderly Research Group. Neurology 2000; 54: S10–15.

54. Andersen K, Launer LJ, Dewey ME et al. Gender differences in the incidence of AD and vascular dementia: The EURODEM Studies. EURODEM Incidence Research Group. Neurology 1999; 53: 1992–7.

55. Kawas C, Gray S, Brookmeyer R, Fozard J, Zonderman A. Age-specific incidence rates of Alzheimer's disease: the Baltimore Longitudinal Study of Aging. Neurology 2000; 54: 2072–7.

56. Shadlen MF, Larson EB, Yukawa M. The epidemiology of Alzheimer's disease and vascular dementia in Japanese and African-American populations: the search for etiological clues. Neurobiol Aging 2000; 21: 171–81.

57. McDowell I. Alzheimer's disease: insights from epidemiology. Aging (Milano) 2001; 13: 143–62.

58. Nussbaum RL, Ellis CE. Alzheimer's disease and Parkinson's disease. N Engl J Med 2003; 348: 1356–64.

59. Evans DA, Hebert LE, Beckett LA et al. Education and other measures of socioeconomic status and risk of incident Alzheimer disease in a defined population of older persons. Arch Neurol 1997; 54: 1399–405.

60. Stern Y, Gurland B, Tatemichi TK et al. Influence of education and occupation on the incidence of Alzheimer's disease. JAMA 1994; 271: 1004–10.

61. Katzman R. Education and the prevalence of dementia and Alzheimer's disease. Neurology 1993; 43: 13–20.

62. Lindsay J, Laurin D, Verreault R et al. Risk factors for Alzheimer's disease: a prospective analysis from the Canadian Study of Health and Aging. Am J Epidemiol 2002; 156: 445–53.

63. Hsiung GY, Sadovnick AD, Feldman H. Apolipoprotein E epsilon4 genotype as a risk factor for cognitive decline and dementia: data from the Canadian Study of Health and Aging. CMAJ 2004; 171: 863–7.

64. Snowdon DA, Kemper SJ, Mortimer JA et al. Linguistic ability in early life and cognitive function and Alzheimer's disease in late life. Findings from the Nun Study. JAMA 1996; 275: 528–32.

65. Whalley LJ, Starr JM, Athawes R et al. Childhood mental ability and dementia. Neurology 2000; 55: 1455–9.

66. Kukull WA, Bowen JD. Dementia epidemiology. Med Clin North Am 2002; 86: 573–90.

67. Scarmeas N, Stern Y. Cognitive reserve and lifestyle. J Clin Exp Neuropsychol 2003; 25: 625–33.

68. van Duijn CM, Clayton D, Chandra V et al. Familial aggregation of Alzheimer's disease and related disorders: a collaborative re-analysis of case-control studies. EURODEM Risk Factors Research Group. Int J Epidemiol 1991; 20 (Suppl 2): S13–20.

69. Green RC, Cupples LA, Go R et al. Risk of dementia among white and African American relatives of patients with Alzheimer disease. JAMA 2002; 287: 329–36.

70. Bird TD. Genetic factors in Alzheimer's disease. N Engl J Med 2005; 352: 862–4.

71. Shobab LA, Hsiung GY, Feldman HH. Cholesterol in Alzheimer's disease. Lancet Neurol 2005; 4: 841–52.

72. Farrer LA, Cupples LA, Haines JL et al. Effects of age, sex, and ethnicity on the association between apolipoprotein E genotype and Alzheimer disease. A meta-analysis. APOE and Alzheimer Disease Meta Analysis Consortium. JAMA 1997; 278: 1349–56.

73. Smith GE, Bohac DL, Waring SC et al. Apolipoprotein E genotype influences cognitive 'phenotype' in patients with Alzheimer's disease but not in healthy control subjects. Neurology 1998; 50: 355–62.

74. Ashford JW, Mortimer JA. Non-familial Alzheimer's disease is mainly due to genetic factors. J Alzheimers Dis 2002; 4: 169–77.

75. Warwick Daw E, Payami H, Nemens EJ et al. The number of trait loci in late-onset Alzheimer disease. Am J Hum Genet 2000; 66: 196–204.

76. Tol J, Roks G, Slooter AJ, van Duijn CM. Genetic and environmental factors in Alzheimer's disease. Rev Neurol (Paris) 1999; 155(Suppl 4): S10–16.

77. Raber J, Huang Y, Ashford JW. ApoE genotype accounts for the vast majority of AD risk and AD pathology. Neurobiol Aging 2004; 25: 641–50.

78. Blacker D, Haines JL, Rodes L et al. ApoE-4 and age at onset of Alzheimer's disease: the NIMH genetics initiative. Neurology 1997; 48: 139–47.

79. Wijsman EM, Daw EW, Yu CE et al. Evidence for a novel late-onset Alzheimer disease locus on chromosome 19p13.2. Am J Hum Genet 2004; 75: 398–409.

80. Liang X, Schnetz-Boutaud N, Kenealy SJ et al. Covariate analysis of late-onset Alzheimer disease refines the chromosome 12 locus. Mol Psychiatry 2006; 11: 280–5.

81. Ertekin-Taner N, Ronald J, Asahara H et al. Fine mapping of the alpha-T catenin gene to a quantitative trait locus on chromosome 10 in late-onset Alzheimer's disease pedigrees. Hum Mol Genet 2003; 12: 3133–43.

82. Myers A, Wavrant De-Vrieze F, Holmans P et al. Full genome screen for Alzheimer disease: stage II analysis. Am J Med Genet 2002; 114: 235–44.

83. Sorbi S, Forleo P, Tedde A et al. Genetic risk factors in familial Alzheimer's disease. Mech Ageing Dev 2001; 122: 1951–60.

CHAPTER 3

The diagnosis of Alzheimer's disease and dementia

Najeeb Qadi and Howard H Feldman

INTRODUCTION

Dementia is the term that describes the loss of prior intellectual capacity within a variety of cognitive domains that can include memory, language, executive function, and visuospatial skills. By definition, this impairment is sufficiently severe to interfere with daily function. Rather than representing a single disease, dementia describes a syndrome that can emerge within >50 diseases.

Alzheimer's disease (AD) is the most common cause of dementia across the lifespan, and its prevalence increases with age.[1] In later life (age >65), it accounts for an estimated 60% of all causes of dementia. Figure 3.1 presents a view of the differential causes of dementia within a national network of dementia research centers, which receives referrals from primary care practitioners.[2]

One of the areas that has been extensively investigated in recent years has been the prodromal state to dementia that is known as mild cognitive impairment (MCI). This condition is elaborated further within this chapter.

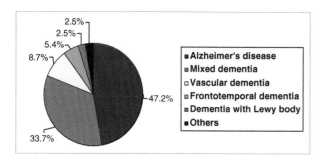

Figure 3.1 The percentages of the different types of dementia. Modified with permission from Feldman et al. A Canadian cohort study of cognitive impairment and related dementias (ACCORD): study methods and baseline results. Neuroepidemiology 2003; 22(5): 265–74.[2]

THE DIAGNOSIS OF ALZHEIMER'S DISEASE

The detection of AD early in its clinical course can be quite challenging, while its identification later in its course is often more obvious. Even one hundred years after Dr Alzheimer's first case of AD, no surrogate biological markers have emerged to definitively diagnose the early stages of this disease. The diagnosis of AD is made clinically at the present time. There are three widely used criteria-based approaches to the diagnosis of AD: the *Diagnostic and Statistical Manual of Mental Disorders*, 4th edition, text revision (DSM-IV-TR) (Table 3.1),[3] the International Classification of Diseases 10th revision (ICD-10),[4] and the National Institute of Neurological and Communicative Disorders and Stroke–Alzheimer's Disease and Related Disorders Association (NINCDS-ADRDA) criteria (Table 3.2).[5]

A number of common clinical features are specified within these three sets of AD diagnostic criteria. Each set of AD criteria requires that patients have cognitive impairment, with memory loss being the central feature of the clinical presentation. They also specify that there should be impairment in at least one other non-memory domain. Other potential causes of dementia need to be excluded, with particular attention paid to exclude delirium. The DSM-IV-TR and ICD-10 criteria require that patients have deficits in activities of daily living or social functioning, whereas the NINCDS-ADRDA criteria leave this point less specified. The differences between the criteria can also be seen in Table 3.3.

In the last several decades, there have been numerous studies examining the sensitivity and specificity of these clinical criteria against the gold standard of

Table 3.1 DSM-IV TR criteria for Alzheimer's disease

A. The development of multiple cognitive deficits manifested by both

   1. Memory impairment (impaired ability to learn new information or to recall previously learned information)

   2. One or more of the following cognitive disturbances:

      (a) aphasia (language disturbance)

      (b) apraxia (impaired ability to carry out motor activities despite intact motor function)

      (c) agnosia (failure to recognize or identify objects despite intact sensory function)

      (d) disturbance in executive functioning (i.e., planning, organizing, sequencing, abstracting)

B. The cognitive deficits in Criteria A1 and A2 each cause significant impairment in social or occupational functioning and represent a significant decline from a previous level of functioning

C. The course is characterized by gradual onset and continuing cognitive decline

D. The cognitive deficits in Criteria A1 and A2 are not due to any of the following:

   1. Other central nervous system conditions that cause progressive deficits in memory and cognition (e.g., cerebrovascular disease, Parkinson's disease, Huntington's disease, subdural hematoma, normal-pressure hydrocephalus, brain tumor)

   2. Systemic conditions that are known to cause dementia (e.g., hypothyroidism, vitamin B or folic acid deficiency, niacin deficiency, hypercalcemia, neurosyphilis, HIV infection)

   3. Substance-induced conditions

E. The deficits do not occur exclusively during the course of a delirium

F. The disturbance is not better accounted for by another Axis I disorder (e.g., Major Depressive Episode, Schizophrenia).

Reproduced with permission from Diagnostic and Statistical Manual of Mental Disorders, 4th edn, text revision. Copyright 2000 American Psychiatric Association.

Table 3.2 NINCDS-ADRDA criteria for Alzheimer's disease

I. Criteria for the clinical diagnosis of PROBABLE AD established by clinical examination and documented by the Mini-Mental Test; Blessed Dementia Scale, or some similar examination, and confirmed by neuropsychological tests;

- deficits in two or more areas of cognition;

- progressive worsening of memory and other cognitive functions;

- no disturbance of consciousness;

- onset between ages 40 and 90, most often after age 65; and

- absence of systemic disorders or other brain diseases that in and of themselves could account for the progressive deficits in memory and cognition

Continued...

Table 3.2 Continued...

II. The diagnosis of PROBABLE AD is supported by:

- progressive deterioration of specific cognitive functions such as language (aphasia), motor skills (apraxia), and perceptions (agnosia);

- impaired activities of daily living and altered patterns of behavior;

- family history of similar disorders, particularly if confirmed neuropathologically; and

- laboratory results of:

  - normal lumbar puncture as evaluated by standard techniques,

  - normal pattern or non-specific changes in EEG, such as increased slow-wave activity, and

  - evidence of cerebral atrophy on CT with progression documented by serial observation

III. Other clinical features consistent with the diagnosis of PROBABLE AD, after exclusion of causes of dementia other than AD, include:

- plateaus in the course of progression of the illness;

- associated symptoms of depression, insomnia, incontinence, delusions, illusions, hallucinations, catastrophic verbal, emotional, or physical outbursts, sexual disorders, and weight loss;

- other neurologic abnormalities in some patients, especially with more advanced disease and including motor signs such as increased muscle tone, myoclonus, or gait disorder;

- seizures in advanced disease; and

- CT normal for age

IV. Features that make the diagnosis of PROBABLE AD uncertain or unlikely include:

- sudden, apoplectic onset;

- focal neurologic findings such as hemiparesis, sensory loss, visual field deficits, and incoordination early in the course of the illness; and

- seizures or gait disturbances at the onset or very early in the course of the illness

Reproduced with permission from McKhann et al. Clinical diagnosis of Alzheimer's disease: report of the NINCDS-ADRDA Work Group under the auspices of Department of Health and Human Services Task Force on Alzheimer's Disease. Neurology 1984; 34(7): 939–44.[5]

Table 3.3 Demonstrating the differences and similarities between the three criteria of AD

Characteristics	ICD-10	DSM-IV	NINCDS-ADRDA Probable AD
Memory decline	+	+	+
Thinking impairment	+	–	–
Aphasia, apraxia, agnosia or disturbed executive function	–	+	–
Impairment of at least one non-memory intellectual function	+	+	+
Dementia established by questionnaire	–	–	+
Dementia confirmed by neuropsychological testing	–	–	+

Continued...

Table 3.3 Continued...

Characteristics	ICD-10	DSM-IV	NINCDS-ADRDA Probable AD
ADL impairment	+	−	−
Social or occupational impairment	−	+	−
Decline from previous level	+	+	+
Onset between age 40 and 90	−	−	+
Insidious onset	+	+	−
Slow deterioration	+	−	+
Continuing deterioration	−	+	+
Absence of clinical or laboratory evidence of another dementing disorder	+	+	+
Absence of sudden onset	+	−	+
Absence of focal neurological signs	+	−	+
Absence of substance abuse	−	+	−
Deficits not limited to delirious period	+	+	+
Absence of another major mental disorder	−	+	−

ICD-10-international Classification of Diseases, 10th revision; DSM-IV-Diagnostic and Statistical Manual of Mental Disorders, 4th edition; NINCDS-ADRDA-National Institute of Neurological and Communicative Disorders and Stroke – Alzheimer's Disease and Related Disorders; AD – Alzheimer's Disease; ADL – activities of daily living. Reproduced with permission from Gauthier S.[6] Clinical Diagnosis and Management of Alzheimer's Disease. 1999.

neuropathologic diagnosis (Table 3.4). In comparing these AD criteria, most studies demonstrate that NINCDS-ADRDA criteria are more sensitive, while the DSM-IV-TR criteria tend to be more specific. With the availability of therapy both for AD and other dementias there has been recognition of the need to improve the specificity of AD diagnosis, which ranges between 60 and 90%. This should be possible in the future with refinement and improvement of neuroimaging and other emerging biological markers. The role of mixed pathologies contributing to dementia in the aging brain allows a more inclusive understanding of the contribution of multiple etiologies. However, criteria for mixed dementia require advancement.

Though AD is the most common dementia, it still must be distinguished from other causes of dementia, including vascular dementia (VaD), frontotemporal dementia (FTD), corticobasal degeneration (CBD), progressive supranuclear palsy (PSP), dementia with Lewy body (DLB), and Parkinson disease dementia (PDD) among others. Prion diseases including Creutzfeld–Jacob

Disease (CJD), Gerstmann–Straussler–Scheinker syndrome (GSS), fatal familial insomnia (FFI), Kuru and Alpers syndrome hold particular significance for their unique patterns of infectivity and related public health considerations.

Treatable causes that can produce dementia include hypothyroidism, syphilis, normal-pressure hydrocephalus (NPH), and nutritional deficiencies such as vitamin B12, folic acid, and thiamine deficiency.

The importance of accurate etiologic diagnosis is underscored by the emerging availability of therapies where longitudinal courses are quite different and genetic implications are quite unique.

Diagnosis in the clinical setting

Essential to an accurate AD clinical diagnosis is a history of both the patient's description of their symptoms as well as an informant's collateral observations. It is vital to obtain a clear history of the temporal profile of the presenting loss of cognitive function, i.e. acute/insidious,

Table 3.4 The sensitivity and specificity of the AD clinical criteria

Study author	Year	NINCDS probable AD sensitivity (%)	NINCDS probable AD specificity (%)	DSM III or DSM IV sensitivity (%)	DSM III or DSM IV specificity (%)
Kukull[7]	1990	92	65	76	80
Jobst[8]	1998	49	100	51	97
Lopez[9]	2000	97	80	—	—
Varma[10]	1999	93	23	—	—
Lim[11]	1999	83	54	—	—
Kazee[12]	1993	98	69	—	—

Reproduced with permission from Varma AR, Snowden JS, Lloyd JJ et al. Evaluation of the NINCDS-ADRDA criteria in the differentiation of Alzheimer's disease and frontotemporal dementia. J Neurol Neurosurg Psychiatry. 1999; 66(2): 184–8.

static/progressive. Typically the AD history is insidious with a gradually progressive course, though occasionally it can start more abruptly. The elucidation of the pattern of cognitive impairment is essential. The memory domain, particularly episodic memory, is the cornerstone of AD diagnosis. Episodic memory refers to the recollection of events with temporal, spatial, and emotional context. Even in the preclinical stages of AD, episodic memory decline can be appreciated.[13] Typically this type of memory impairment is the leading presenting symptom of AD. On bedside testing, AD patients have decreased delayed recall on new learning tasks and impaired learning curves.[14] They also perform poorly when given semantic or categoric cueing. There is usually a temporal gradient in memory impairment where shorter-term memory is more impaired than longer-term, yet both decline as the disease advances. Semantic memory, which refers to the memory of the meaning of words and other factual knowledge, is also impaired in AD. There is relative preservation of procedural memory, the system that allows motor learning, until the late stages of the illness.

Beyond memory deficits, executive dysfunction is most typically the second cognitive domain to become impaired. It also leads patients to cross the diagnostic line from MCI to dementia, as their social function and activities of daily living are affected. Executive impairment can include motivation, strategy development and adjustment, response control, and abstraction. These functions are mediated primarily by frontal cortical and subcortical brain regions.[15] In AD, executive functional impairment unfolds slowly and progressively.

THE DIFFERENTIAL DIAGNOSIS OF DEMENTIA (TABLE 3.5)

Several important differential diagnoses of AD are described here.

Neurodegenerative disorders

Pick complex

This term has emerged to describe a group of neurodegenerative disorders that include the frontal/temporal, parietal, and subcortical structures.[17] It has been alternatively referred to as frontotemporal lobar degeneration or simply FTD. However, the broader term seems to better capture the spectrum of related conditions including (a)–(d).

(a) Frontotemporal degeneration (FTD)

There are three distinct clinical syndromes recognized within FTD where there is focal degeneration of frontal/temporal lobes:[18]

- The frontal behavioral variant, which includes individuals with prominent changes in social behavior and personality.

- Semantic dementia, which is characterized by a loss of semantic memory with frequent visual associative losses.

- Progressive non-fluent aphasia in which the phonologic and syntactic components of language are affected.

Characteristic features that help to distinguish FTD from AD include concreteness of thought, echolalia, perseverative

Table 3.5   Differential diagnosis of dementia

Degenerative

Alzheimer's disease

Pick complex

- FTD
- CBD
- PSP
- FTD-MND

Dementia with Lewy bodies

Parkinson disease dementia

Multiple system atrophy

Huntington's disease

Vascular dementia

Multiple infarction

Strategic infarction

Multi-lacunar state leukoencephalopathy

Subcortical ischemic encephalopathy

Post subarachnoid hemorrhage

Cerebral autosomal dominant arteriopathy with subcortical infarcts and leukoencephalopathy

Cerebral angiitis

Anoxic brain injury

Genetic

Adrenoleukodystrophy

Dentatorubropallidoluysian atrophy

Mitochondrial disorders (MERFF, MELAS, Leighs)

Niemann Pick type C

Spinocerebellar ataxia

Tumor

Glioblastoma multiforme

Primary CNS lymphoma

Metastatic tumor

Paraneoplastic-limbic encephalitis

CNS Infection

TB meningitis

Fungal meningitis

Syphilis

AIDS dementia

Prion diseases

Post herpes simplex encephalitis

Psychiatric

Depression

Alcohol abuse

Drug use or abuse

Schizophrenia

Bipolar disease

Trauma

Subdural hematoma

Closed head injury

Open head injury

Dementia pugilistica

Toxic/metabolic

B12 deficiency

Folate deficiency

Hyperhomocysteinemia

Thyroid deficiency

Multisystem failure

Heavy metal toxicity

Other toxic exposure, e.g. glue,

Other

Normal-pressure hydrocephalus

Modified with permission from Neill R.[16] Graff-Radford. Alzheimer's Disease Jacksonville Medicine. February, 2000.

responses, and stereotyped use of words and phrases. Mutism ensues in the course of these disorders.[19] Spatial skills are relatively preserved early, a distinguishing feature between FTD and AD.

(b) Corticobasal degeneration (CBD)

This disorder is characterized by atrophy of multiple brain regions including the cerebral cortex and the basal ganglia. Initial symptoms first appear with marked asymmetric apraxia, though eventually both sides are affected as the disease progresses. Motor symptoms include poor coordination, akinesia (an absence of movements), rigidity (a resistance to imposed movement), disequilibrium (impaired balance), limb dystonia (abnormal muscle postures), and myoclonus (muscular jerks). The cognitive profile includes visuospatial impairment, apraxia (loss of the ability to make familiar, purposeful movements), and dysarthria with hesitant and halting speech. The alien hand syndrome in which the patient does not recognize his hand as being part of his own body is quite characteristic for CBD.[20]

(c) Progressive supranuclear palsy (PSP)

This degenerative illness is characterized by vertical supranuclear palsy with prominent postural instability and falls, often even in the first year following onset. The cognitive profile includes slowed cognitive processing, sequencing and planning difficulties, mild memory difficulty, and apathy. Cognitive dysfunction and personality change are generally milder in degree compared to AD.[21]

(d) Frontotemporal dementia – motor neuron disease (FTD-MND)

A great deal of interest has been shown in the association of dementia with MND. There are cases of FTD developing MND, as well as MND associated with a frontal type of dementia. In this subtype, the dementia is associated weakness, muscle atrophy, and myoclonus, the cardinal features of MND. The dementia in this subtype can have behavioral and/or language changes seen in other subtypes of FTD.[22]

Dementia with Lewy bodies (DLB)/Parkinson disease dementia (PDD)

There is a spectrum of dementia that occurs with the presence of Lewy bodies and α-synuclein aggregation in the brain. Clinically, the disorders are described as DLB and PDD. The timing of motor symptom onset is currently used to differentiate PDD from DLB.[23] In DLB, the motor parkinsonism occurs at or near the onset of cognitive decline, while in PDD, the dementia develops typically years after the diagnosis of PD. The core features of DLB include spontaneous motor parkinsonism, fluctuating cognition with pronounced variations in attention and alertness, and recurrent well-formed and detailed visual hallucinations. The important supportive symptoms of both DLB and PDD include REM sleep behavioral disorder and severe neuroleptic sensitivity.[23] In REM sleep, behavioral disorder sleep paralysis, which normally disables the voluntary muscles during REM sleep, fails to occur. The result is that the sufferer acts out movements that occur in dreams, sometimes with injurious results. From the cognitive standpoint, in DLB, memory impairment is often not as prominent at

diagnosis as in AD, whereas deficits in attention, visuospatial ability, and executive function are more prominent.[24]

Vascular dementia (VaD)

This condition results from cerebrovascular injury that produces vascular cognitive impairment. It is the second most common cause of dementia when it is associated with AD.[25] However, in its pure form, it is an infrequent cause of dementia. The presentation and cause of vascular dementia are determined by the location and timing of vascular injury, as well as the nature of the vascular injury. Individuals with VaD may have multiple infarctions involving large areas of cortex, strategic infarcts in areas such as the thalamus, hippocampus, or parietal lobes, or subcortical vascular dementia related to ischemic leukoencephalopathy. Combinations of these mechanisms can occur causing significant heterogeneity. A common cognitive pattern in VaD includes prominent executive dysfunction, suggestive of frontal involvement.[26] Given these disparate mechanisms of injury, generalizations are limited. However, the onset and course of VaD typically differs from AD. Whereas the onset in AD is insidious and gradual, VaD has stepwise decline or progressive decline with highlighting brief downturns.

Normal-pressure hydrocephalus (NPH)

This disorder attracts considerable interest in the differential diagnosis of AD, as it is potentially treatable with neurosurgical shunting of cerebrospinal fluid (CSF). The classic clinical presentation of NPH is one of progressive gait apraxia, urinary incontinence, and dementia. Patients with NPH show subcortical cognitive deficits including forgetfulness, decreased attention, inertia, and bradyphrenia; the progression is less rapid than the dementia of AD.[27] Patients also do not present with the 'aphasia–apraxia–agnosia syndrome', which is typical for cortical dementia, e.g. AD.

Creutzfeld–Jacob disease

Prion diseases, particularly sporadic CJD and variant CJD, often present with an unusually rapid course and progression over weeks to months rather than years.[28] Probable CJD disease is diagnosed by the WHO criteria when patients have rapidly progressive dementia, periodic sharp waves in the EEG, and at least two of the following: myoclonus, visual and/or cerebellar symptoms, pyramidal and/or extrapyramidal signs, and akinetic mutism.

The initial clinical assessment is complemented by laboratory studies that should include a complete blood count, electrolytes, urinalysis, B12 and folate levels, and thyroid function tests. Structural neuroimaging with computerized tomography (CT) head scan or magnetic resonance imaging (MRI) assists in identifying comorbid diseases. Supplementary tests including lumber puncture for CSF analysis, further functional neuroimaging, and genetic investigations can be selectively helpful.

ADVANCES IN NEUROIMAGING

A variety of neuroimaging approaches have been developed that allow non-invasive imaging of the brain's structure and function. Structural neuroimaging includes CT and MRI, while functional neuroimaging includes magnetic resonance spectroscopy (MRS), single photon emission computed tomography (SPECT), positron emission tomography (PET), and functional MRI (fMRI). These techniques are increasingly available and offer prospects for improving the accuracy of diagnosis of dementia, achieving earlier diagnosis, following the course of the disease, and capturing response to therapy. Familiarization with the technologies, their potential, and their limitations is germane to both the clinical care and to clinical research.

STRUCTURAL IMAGING

A set of evidence-based consensus criteria for CT neuroimaging in dementia in primary care is presented in Table 3.6.[29] CT brain imaging was pioneered in the 1970s, allowing the first visualization of the brain parenchyma. Its early use in dementia was directed at

Table 3.6 Criteria for performing CT head scan

1. Age less than 60 years

2. Rapid (e.g., over 1 to 2 months) unexplained decline in cognition or function

3. Short duration of dementia (less than 2 years)

4. Recent/significant head trauma

5. Unexplained neurologic symptoms (e.g., new onset of severe headache or seizures)

6. History of cancer (especially in sites and types that metastasize to the brain)

7. Use of anticoagulants or history of a bleeding disorder

8. History of urinary incontinence and gait disorder early in the course of dementia (as may be found in normal pressure hydrocephalus)

9. Any new localizing sign (e.g., hemiparesis or a Babinski reflex)

10. Unusual or atypical cognitive symptoms or presentation (e.g., progressive aphasia)

11. Gait disturbance

Reproduced with permission from Patterson C et al. The recognition, assessment and management of dementing disorders: conclusions from the Canadian Consensus Conference on Dementia. Can J Neurol Sci. 2001; 28 (Suppl 1): S3–16.[29]

excluding conditions that might be amenable to neuro-surgical treatment, though the yield of this procedure in finding this type of problem has proven to be very low (<1%). See Figure 3.2.

In the past two decades, MRI has been introduced and has matured to provide higher resolution of brain

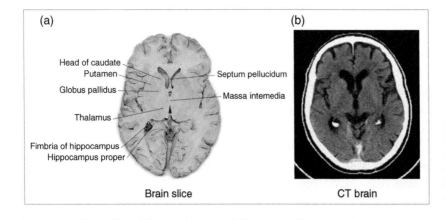

Figure 3.2 Axial view of the brain. (a) Brain slice. (b) CT image. Reproduced with permission from Brain slice: www.indiana.edu/~m555/axial/axial.html) and CT brain: imaginis.com/graphics/ct-scan/Image40.jpg.

structures than CT. It better visualizes the white matter, identifies vascular lesions, and detects other pathologic disturbances. It has become the preferred technique for detailed structural neuroimaging. MRI does not use ionizing radiation and therefore reduces the cumulative radiation burden.[30] MRI access is less prevalent than CT, with more limited availability in some countries, which restricts access. See Figures 3.3 and 3.4.

While the neuroimaging detection of the hallmark microscopic pathologic changes of senile plaques (SNPs) and neurofibrillary tangles (NFTs) remains elusive, the related changes in the brain that result in volume loss and atrophy can now be measured increasingly accurately using MRI. AD whole brain volumes declined by 2.4 + 1.4% compared to 0.4 + 0.7% in normal subjects, when two MRI scans with a mean interscan period of

1.8 years were performed.[32] This has stimulated considerable interest in trying to develop these types of techniques for clinical use.

When the duration of illness and AD stage are taken into account, the volumetric loss within the hippocampus best discriminates between patients with AD in its early stages and normal controls. As the disease progresses, volume loss occurs within the anterior cingulate, the inferior and medial temporal lobes, the basal ganglia, and the amygdala. Hence, in keeping with the neuropathologic evolution of the disease, these findings fit well with the longitudinal observations that there is hippocampal atrophy early in the disease and more widespread volume loss later.[33] These patterns may be particularly important in predicting conversion of MCI to AD. When normal individuals are compared with those having MCI who

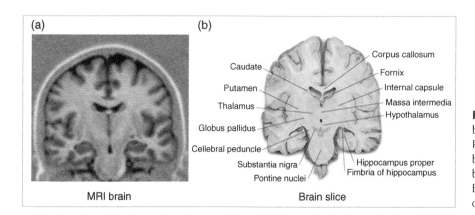

(a)   (b)

Caudate
Putamen
Thalamus
Globus pallidus
Cellebral peduncle
Substantia nigra
Pontine nuclei

Corpus callosum
Fornix
Internal capsule
Massa intermedia
Hypothalamus

Hippocampus proper
Fimbria of hippocampus

MRI brain   Brain slice

Figure 3.3 Coronal view of the brain. (a) MRI image. (b) Brain slice. Reproduced with permission from MRI brain: www.mrtip.com/exam_gifs/brain_mri_inversion_recover.gif, and Brain slice:www.indiana.edu/~m555/coron/coron.html.

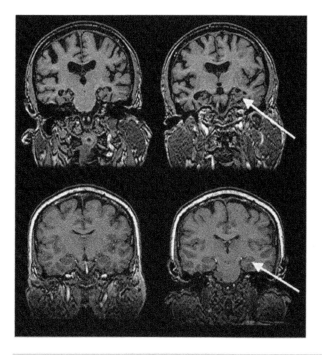

Figure 3.4 MR images of a patient with AD (above) and in a normal aged subject (below). These images show generalized atrophy in AD and also considerable hippocampal atrophy in the AD subject but not in the normal subject (arrows). Reproduced with permission from Tomaszewski et al. Clinical Neuroscience. Research. 2004; 3: 383–395.[31]

progress to AD, the accuracy of discrimination is 93% based on the MRI cortical measurements of the entorhinal cortex, banks of the superior temporal sulcus, and anterior portion of the cingulate sulcus. However, only 75% accuracy is found in discriminating MCI subjects who within 3 years of follow-up either develop AD or remain stable.[34] The volume of the entorhinal cortex may differentiate individuals who will develop dementia with greater accuracy than hippocampal measures.[35] See Figure 3.5.

FUNCTIONAL IMAGING

SPECT and PET

SPECT and PET are techniques that use radionuclide isotopes to allow *in vivo* imaging of brain metabolism and blood flow. They have been advancing steadily from their introduction, though still have had limited clinical application. See Figures 3.6 and 3.7. PET was the first neuroimaging technique to be used to study cerebral activation. 18Fluorodeoxyglucose (18FDG) PET

provides a map of glucose metabolism, an essential neuronal function, over a period of time.[39]

Studies in AD using 18FDG PET have shown that the most characteristic pattern found in early AD is decreased metabolism bilaterally in the parietotemporal association cortex and cingulate gyrus.[36] It has also been possible to show a benefit in medial temporal lobe metabolism 3 months after the administration of cholinesterase inhibitors (ChEIs) using FDG.[40] See Figure 3.8. This may hold the potential to become a surrogate marker, however it is still too costly and inaccessible for regular clinical use.

PET has also been used in conjugation with [(11)C]PK 11195, a ligand that binds to microglia, to demonstrate microglial activation in AD in a pattern consistent with the location of senile plaques seen in post-mortem histopathology.[41]

Recently, it has become possible to visualize aggregating AD proteins *in vivo*. Ligands including 2-(1-{6-[(2-fluoroethyl)(methyl)amino]-2-naphthyl}ethylidene) malononitrile (FDDNP)[42] and Pittsburgh compound B (PIB)[43] have been developed. These ligands enable greater accuracy in the diagnosis and evaluation of the

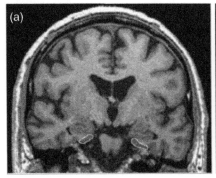
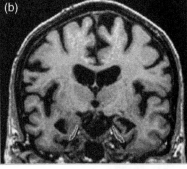

Figure 3.5 Coronal MRI at the level of the mammillary bodies. The entorhinal cortex has been outlined in a normal control (a) and a person with mild cognitive impairment (b). Reproduced with permission from Masdeu et al. Neuroimaging as a marker of the onset and progression of Alzheimer's disease. Journal of the Neurological Sciences 2005; 236: 55–64.[36]

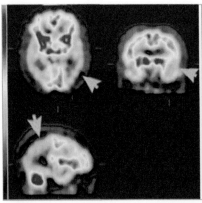
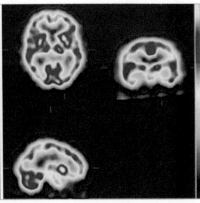

Figure 3.6 99m-Tc HMPAO SPECT (AD vs depression). Left image (51 y, m): symmetric hypoperfusion temporoparietal regions (shown by arrows) in a patient with AD. Right image (73 y, m): almost normal brain perfusion in a patient with depression. Reproduced with permission from Mirzaei et al. Current Alzheimer Research 2004; 1: 219–29.[37]

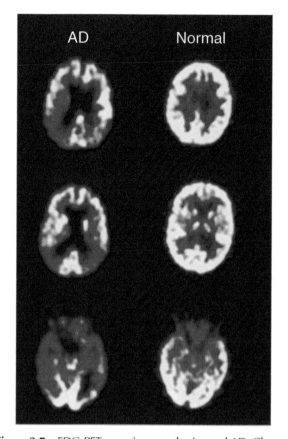

Figure 3.7 FDG-PET scans in normal aging and AD. Glucose metabolism is presented on a heat scale, with brighter colors reflecting greater glucose utilization. Glucose metabolism is reduced in posterior cortical regions (temporal and parietal lobes) in patients with AD. Modified with permission from Jagust W. NeuroRx. 2004; 1(2): 206–12.[38]

benefit of therapeutic interventions in the accumulation of abnormal proteins. See Figure 3.9.

There is a marked retention of PIB in the association cortices in AD where there are large numbers of SNPs and NFTs. PIB is proposed to have specificity for labeling of amyloid plaques while FDDNP likely does have this same specificity. By contrast, retention is equal in AD patients and controls in areas known to be relatively unaffected by amyloid deposition (such as the subcortical white matter, pons, and cerebellum).[45] See Figure 3.10.

SPECT is cheaper than PET and more widely available within most nuclear departments. It is reported to have less sensitivity and specificity than PET for early AD diagnosis. The two labels most used for SPECT are technetium, mostly for hexamethyl propylene-amine-oxime (HMPAO)[47] studies of cerebral blood flow, and iodine for receptor ligand studies (muscarinic, dopamine D2, benzodiazepine).[48]

MRI

Magnetic resonance spectroscopy

Magnetic resonance spectroscopy (MRS) allows the non-invasive quantitation of a number of chemical compounds important for brain function. The concentration of phosphodiesters has been associated with the amount of

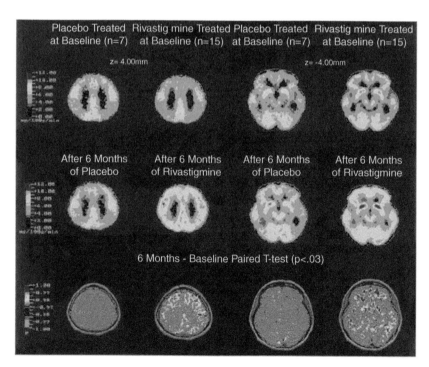

Figure 3.8 Absolute glucose metabolism (mg/100 g/min) in rivastigmine responders and placebo-treated patients at baseline and following 6 months' treatment. Reproduced with permission from Potkin et al. Brain metabolic and clinical effects of rivastigmine in Alzheimer's disease. International Journal of Neuropsychopharmacology 2001: (4) 223–230.[40] Cambridge University Press.

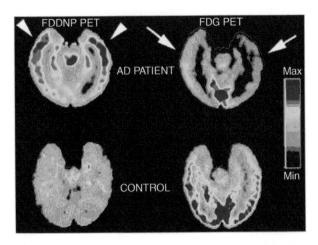

Figure 3.9 PET images comparing temporal lobe uptake of [18F] FDDNP, an amyloid binding radiotracer, and FDG, a marker of glucose metabolism, in a patient with AD (left) and a control subject (right). Note increased uptake and retention of [18F] FDDNP (arrowheads) in temporal lobes of the patient with AD, compared with those in control subject. Reproduced with permission from Petrella et al. Neuroimaging and early diagnosis of Alzheimer's disease: a look to the future. Radiology 2003; 226: 315–36.[44]

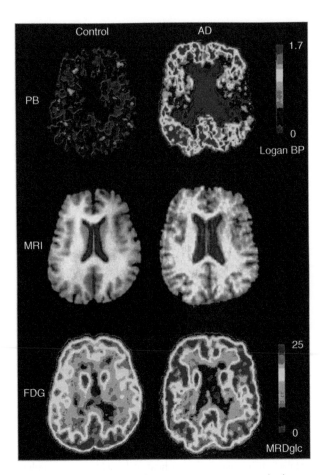

Figure 3.10 Compound B (PIB) (top row) and glucose metabolism (bottom row) measured in a 70-year-old healthy control subject and a 75-year-old subject with AD. Also shown is the corresponding anatomic MRI (middle row). Greater retention of PIB is evident in frontal, temporoparietal, and posterior cingulate cortices, and less PIB retention is evident in the sensory-motor strip of the AD subject, relative to the control. Reproduced with permission from Chester et al. Arch Neurol 2005; 62: 196–200.[46]

amyloid plaques. Reduced levels of *N*-acetylaspartate (NAA) are considered a sensitive marker of neuronal damage or loss. The recovery of NAA levels predicts clinical improvement or slowing of cognitive decline. A combination of atrophy-corrected NAA level and MRI-measured atrophy has been reported to have a better than 90% discrimination of AD from control subjects.[49] In AD, NAA levels decline in parallel with cognitive function, and have been shown to increase in response to cholinesterase inhibitor treatment. See Figure 3.11. This technique is still technically challenging, with signal/noise problems and difficulty with its broad implementation.

Functional MRI

Functional MRI (fMRI) uses specialized MRI pulse sequences to study *in vivo* cognitive function. This technique was developed in the 1990s and is evolving rapidly. It uses blood oxygen level dependent contrast to map brain activity during sensory and cognitive stimulation. Cognitive activation paradigms which are sensitive to early damage changes in AD are being developed at present.

For example in AD, studying the function of the medial temporal lobe (MTL) in response to memory activation tasks may permit the identification of functional abnormalities that precede atrophy. A clinical study

reported diminished activation in the MTL in AD patients compared with controls and also diminished entorhinal activation in 4 of the 12 MCI patients, in early AD.[51] fMRI is both a challenging and promising development, because it combines structural and functional aspects in one technique, with high temporal and spatial resolution, and lacks some of the disadvantages of PET. Much work still remains to be done with fMRI, before it is clinically accessible. See Figure 3.12.

Magnetization transfer imaging

Magnetization transfer imaging (MTI) maps the density of macromolecules in tissue. It has been shown in inflammatory white matter diseases to be a strong

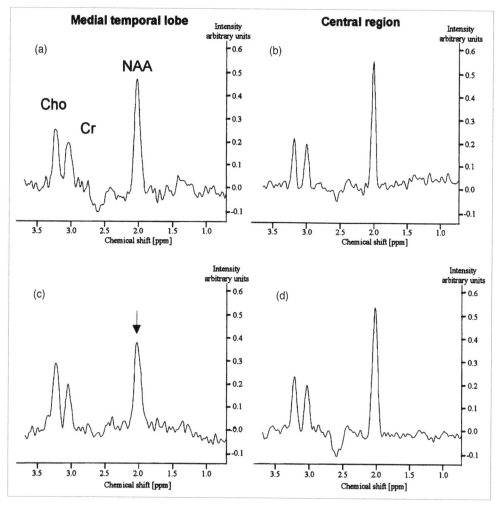

Figure 3.11 Proton MR spectra of a healthy 71-year-old control subject (a, b) and a 77-year-old patient with AD (c, d). The arrow in panel (c) points to the reduced N-acetylaspartate (NAA) peak in the AD patient. Cho = choline; Cr = creatine/phosphocreatine. Reproduced with permission from Jessen et al. Neurology 2000; 55(5): 684–8.[50]

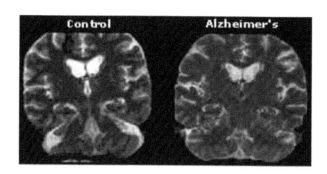

Figure 3.12 Acute oxidative metabolism is measured using fMRI to see where the brain fires when it is performing an activation task. Here, subjects tried to memorize a series of faces shown to them, and the resulting activation in the hippocampus was lower in Alzheimer's patients. Modified with permission from Small et al. Differential regional dysfunction of the hippocampal formation among elderly with memory decline and Alzheimer's disease. Annals of Neurology 1999; 45(4): 466–72.[51]

predictor of the severity of neuropsychologic deficits.[52] MTI requires extensive post-processing to generate clinically useful data and has uncertain benefit in AD.

Diffusion tensor imaging

Diffusion tensor imaging (DTI) provides a visualization of the location, the orientation, and directional dependence (anisotropy) of the brain's white matter tracts. Therefore, it can allow a visualization of the integrity of the white matter tracts. Although AD pathology mainly affects cortical gray matter, MRI studies have shown that changes also exist in the white matter. A recent study has revealed abnormalities in the frontal and temporal white matter in early AD patients, changes that are compatible with early temporal-to-frontal disconnections.[53] See Figures 3.13 and 3.14.

BIOMARKERS FOR AD

There is no currently available diagnostic biomarker for either the diagnosis or monitoring of the course of AD. This has been a major impediment to the investigation of disease modifying therapies, but one that may foreseeably be resolved. There is currently significant interest in cerebrospinal fluid (CSF) measurement of tau and β-amyloid in their various forms.

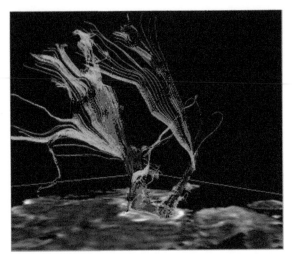

Figure 3.13 DTI visualizing axonal pathways. Reproduced with permission from Philipp Staempfli, Thomas Jaermann, Peter Boesiger, Institute for Biomedical Engineering, University and ETH Zurich and Spyros Kollias Institute for Neuroradiology, University Hospital Zurich.

Cerebrospinal fluid markers

Through monitoring of CSF tau and β-amyloid, it may be possible to monitor the neuropathologic footprint of AD.

The use of CSF assays to predict the diagnosis of AD has been suggested on the basis of the findings that low levels of CSF Aβ 1–42 and high levels of CSF total tau (T-tau) have been found both in early AD and in patients with MCI who later convert to AD.[54] The elevated CSF levels of T-tau in AD in later stages predict severe neurodegeneration.[55] However, the finding of elevated CSF levels of phosphorylated tau (P-tau) in AD has been suggested to represent hyperphosphorylation of tau and formation of NFT.[56] This finding may be specific for AD as normal levels of P-tau are found in patients with other types of dementia.[57]

How the levels of these CSF biomarkers reflect the severity of symptoms or disease progression in AD is still under investigation. However, it is important to recognize that currently CSF biomarkers in isolation are insufficient to diagnose or exclude AD. They must be interpreted in light of all of the clinical, neuropsychologic, other laboratory, and neuroimaging data available. See Figure 3.15.

Blood

Given its accessibility, the monitoring of biomarkers in blood in AD is attractive. Blood is easier to obtain and has fewer side-effects than spinal fluid testing. More recently, there has been growing interest in measuring

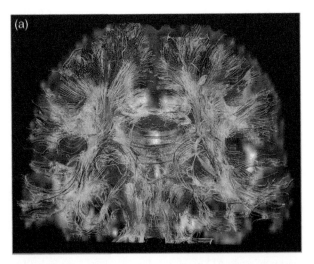
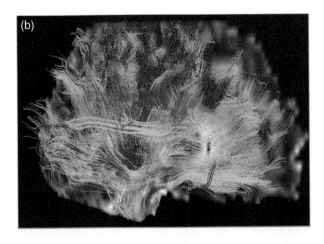

Figure 3.14 DTI visualizing axonal pathways in a whole brain: coronal view (a) and saggital view (b). Reproduced with permission from Thomas Jaermann, Philipp Staempfli, Peter Boesiger. Institute for Biomedical Engineering, University and ETH Zurich and Spyros Kollias Institute for Neuroradiology, University Hospital Zurich.

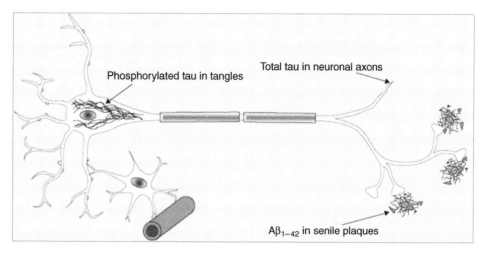

Figure 3.15   Schematic drawing of a neuron with an adjacent astrocyte and capillary. The central pathogenetic processes in AD and their corresponding biochemical markers are depicted. Total concentration of tau protein is a marker of neuronal and axonal degeneration, $A\beta_{1-42}$ concentration is a marker of plaque formation, and concentration of phosphorylated tau is a marker for hyperphosphorylation of tau and formation of tangles. Reproduced with permission from Blennow K, Hampel H. Lancet Neurology 2003; 2(10): 605–13.[58]

isoprostanes in blood and CSF. Isoprostanes are prostaglandin-like compounds that are produced by free radical mediated peroxidation of lipoproteins, a process that may be injurious to neurons.[59]

Markers of inflammation (C-reactive protein, tumor necrosis factor, interleukin) and metabolism (insulin degrading enzyme, growth hormone, cortisol, and other steroids) have been reported to correlate with clinical findings of aging and cognitive decline.

CONCLUSION

Dementia is a condition in which there is impairment within a variety of cognitive domains that are sufficiently severely affected as to interfere with daily function. AD, the most common cause of dementia, is diagnosed clinically at present. Though there are over 50 other causes of dementia, AD can be relatively recognized by its clinical phenotype and supported by neuroimaging and selected biomarker testing. Both structural and functional neuroimaging can support the clinical diagnosis of AD and may in the future play a major part in establishing the diagnosis on their own. There is a growing interest in CSF markers as they define the footprint of neurodegeneration in AD.

REFERENCES

1. Ritchie K, Kildea D, Robine JM. The relationship between age and the prevalence of senile dementia: a meta-analysis of recent data. Int J Epidemiol 1992; 21(4): 763–9.
2. Feldman H, Levy AR, Hsiung GY et al. A Canadian cohort study of cognitive impairment and related dementias (ACCORD): study methods and baseline results. Neuroepidemiology 2003; 22(5): 265–74.
3. American Psychiatric Association. Diagnostic and Statistical Manual of Mental Disorders, 4th edn, text revision. Washington, DC: American Psychiatric Association, 2000.
4. World Health Organization. The ICD-10 Classification of Mental and Behavioural Disorders. Geneva: World Health Organization, 1992.
5. McKhann G, Drachman D, Folstein M et al. Clinical diagnosis of Alzheimer's disease: report of the NINCDS-ADRDA Work Group under the auspices of Department of Health and Human Services Task Force on Alzheimer's Disease. Neurology 1984; 34(7): 939–44.
6. Gauthier S. Clinical Diagnosis and Management of Alzheimer's Disease 1999.
7. Kukull WA, Larson EB, Reifler BV et al. The validity of 3 clinical diagnostic criteria for Alzheimer's disease. Neurology 1990; 40(9): 1364–9.
8. Jobst KA, Barnetson LP, Shepstone BJ. Accurate prediction of histologically confirmed Alzheimer's disease and the differential diagnosis of dementia: the use of NINCDS-ADRDA and DSM-III-R criteria, SPECT, X-ray CT, and Apo E4 in medial temporal lobe dementias. Oxford Project to Investigate Memory and Aging. Int Psychogeriatr 1998; 10(3): 271–302.

9. Lopez OL, Becker JT, Klunk W et al. Research evaluation and diagnosis of probable Alzheimer's disease over the last two decades: I. Neurology 2000; 55(12): 1854–62.

10. Varma

11. Lim A, Tsuang D, Kukull W et al. Clinico-neuropathological correlation of Alzheimer's disease in a community-based case series. J Am Geriatr Soc. 1999; 47(5): 564–9.

12. Kazee AM, Eskin TA, Lapham LW et al. Clinico-pathologic correlates in Alzheimer disease: assessment of clinical and pathologic diagnostic criteria. Alzheimer Dis Assoc Disord 1993; 7(3): 152–64.

13. Backman L, Small BJ, Fratiglioni L. Stability of the pre-clinical episodic memory deficit in Alzheimer's disease. Brain 2001; 124(Pt 1): 96–102.

14. Chen P, Ratcliff G, Belle SH et al. Cognitive tests that best discriminate between presymptomatic AD and those who remain nondemented. Neurology 2000; 55(12): 1847–53.

15. Case R. The role of the frontal lobes in the regulation of cognitive development. Brain Cogn 1992; 20(1): 51–73.

16. Neill R

17. Kertesz A, Davidson W, Munoz DG. Clinical and pathological overlap between frontotemporal dementia, primary progressive aphasia and corticobasal degeneration: the Pick complex. Dement Geriatr Cogn Disord 1999; 10(Suppl 1): 46–9.

18. Snowden JS, Neary D, Mann DMA. Frontotemporal Lobar Degeneration: Frontotemporal Dementia, Progressive Aphasia, Semantic Dementia. London: Churchill Livingstone, 1996.

19. Bozeat S, Gregory CA, Ralph MA, Hodges JR. Which neuropsychiatric and behavioural features distinguish frontal and temporal variants of frontotemporal dementia from Alzheimer's disease? J Neurol Neurosurg Psychiatry 2000; 69(2): 178–86.

20. Lang AE, Bergeron C, Pollanen MS et al. Parietal Pick's disease mimicking cortical-basal ganglionic degeneration. Neurology 1994; 44(8): 1436–40.

21. Litvan I, Mangone CA, McKee A et al. Natural history of progressive supranuclear palsy Steele–Richardson–Olszewski syndrome) and clinical predictors of survival: a clinicopathological study. J Neurol Neurosurg Psychiatry 1996; 60(6): 615–20.

22. Neary D, Snowden JS, Mann DM. Cognitive change in motor neurone disease/amyotrophic lateral sclerosis (MND/ALS). J Neurol Sci 2000; 180(1–2): 15–20.

23. McKeith IG, Dickson DW, Lowe J et al. Diagnosis and management of dementia with Lewy bodies: third report of the DLB Consortium. Neurology 2005; 65(12): 1863–72.

24. Simard M, van Reekum R, Cohen T. A review of the cognitive and behavioral symptoms in dementia with Lewy bodies. J Neuropsychiatry Clin Neurosci 2000; 12(4): 425–50.

25. Canadian study of health and aging: study methods and prevalence of dementia. CMAJ 1994; 150(6): 899–913.

26. Villardita C. Alzheimer's disease compared with cerebro-vascular dementia. Neuropsychological similarities and differences. Acta Neurol Scand 1993; 87(4): 299–308.

27. Vanneste JA. Diagnosis and management of normal-pressure hydrocephalus. J Neurol 2000; 247(1): 5–14.

28. Brown P, Gibbs CJ Jr, Rodgers-Johnson P et al. Human spongiform encephalopathy: the National Institutes of Health series of 300 cases of experimentally transmitted disease. Ann Neurol 1994; 35(5): 513–29.

29. Patterson C, Gauthier S, Bergman H et al. The recognition, assessment and management of dementing disorders: conclusions from the Canadian Consensus Conference on Dementia. Can J Neurol Sci 2001; 28(Suppl 1): S3–16.

30. Kent DL, Haynor DR, Longstreth WT Jr et al. The clinical efficacy of magnetic resonance imaging in neuroimaging. Ann Intern Med 1994; 120(10): 856–71.

31. Tomaszewski Farias S, Jagust WJ. Neuroimaging in non-Alzheimer dementias. Clinical Neuroscience Research 2004; 3: 383–95.

32. Fox NC, Scahill RI, Crum WR et al. Correlation between rates of brain atrophy and cognitive decline in AD. Neurology 1999; 52: 1687–9.

33. Pennanen C, Kivipelto M, Tuomainen S et al. Hippocampus and entorhinal cortex in mild cognitive impairment and early AD. Neurobiol Aging 2004; 25(3): 303–10.

34. Killiany RJ, Gomez-Isla T, Moss M et al. Use of structural magnetic resonance imaging to predict who will get Alzheimer's disease. Ann Neurol 2000; 47: 430–9.

35. Killiany RJ, Hyman BT, Gomez-Isla T et al. MRI measures of entorhinal cortex vs. hippocampus in preclinical AD. Neurology 2002; 58: 1188–96.

36. Masdeu JC, Zubieta JL, Arbizu J. Neuroimaging as a marker of the onset and progression of Alzheimer's disease. J Neurol Sci 2005; 236(1–2): 55–64.

37. Mirzaei S, Gelpi E, Booij J et al. New approaches in nuclear medicine for early diagnosis of Alzheimer's disease. Curr Alzheimer Res 2004; 1(3): 219–29.

38. Jagust W. NeuroRx 2004; 1(2): 206–12.

39. Sokoloff L. Localization of functional activity in the central nervous system by measurement of glucose utilization with radioactive deoxyglucose. J Cereb Blood Flow Metab 1981; 1(1): 7–36.

40. Potkin SG, Anand R, Fleming K et al. Brain metabolic and clinical effects of rivastigmine in Alzheimer's disease. Int J Neuropsychopharmacol 2001; 4(3): 223–30.

41. Cagnin A, Brooks DJ, Kennedy AM et al. In-vivo measurement of activated microglia in dementia. Lancet 2001; 358: 461–7.

42. Shoghi-Jadid K, Small GW, Agdeppa ED et al. Localization of neurofibrillary tangles and beta-amyloid plaques in the brains of living patients with Alzheimer disease. Am J Geriatr Psychiatry 2002; 10: 24–35.

43. Mathis CA, Wang Y, Holt DP et al. Synthesis and evaluation of 11C-labeled 6-substituted 2-arylbenzothiazoles as amyloid imaging agents. J Med Chem 2003; 46: 2740–54.

44. Petrella JR, Coleman RE, Doralswamy PM. Neuroimaging and early diagnosis of Alzheimer's disease: a look to the future. Radiology 2003; 226: 315–36.

45. Klunk WE, Engler H, Nordberg A et al. Imaging brain amyloid in Alzheimer's disease with Pittsburgh Compound-B. Ann Neurol 2004; 55: 306–19.

46. Mathis CA, Klunk WE, Price JC et al. Imaging technology for neurodegenerative diseases: progress toward detection of specific pathologies. Arch Neurol 2005; 62: 196–200.

47. Momose T, Kosaka N, Nishikawa J et al. A new method for brain functional study using Tc-99m HMPAO SPECT. Radiat Med 1989; 7(2): 82–7.

48. Costa DC, Verhoeff NP, Cullum ID et al. In vivo characterisation of 3-iodo-6-methoxybenzamide 123I in humans. Eur J Nucl Med 1990; 16(11): 813–16.

49. Schuff N, Capizzano AA, Du AT et al. Selective reduction of N-acetylaspartate in medial temporal and parietal lobes in AD. Neurology 2002; 58: 928–35.

50. Jesson F, Block W, Traber F et al. Proton MR spectroscopy detects a relative decrease of N-acetylaspartate in the medial temporal lobe of patients with AD. Neurology 2000; 55(5): 684–8.

51. Small SA, Perera GM, DeLaPaz R et al. Differential regional dysfunction of the hippocampal formation among elderly with memory decline and Alzheimer's disease. Ann Neurol 1999; 45: 466–72.

52. van Buchem MA, Grossman RI, Armstrong C, Polansky M et al. Correlation of volumetric magnetization transfer imaging with clinical data in MS. Neurology 1998; 50(6): 1609–17.

53. Naggara O, Oppenheim C, Rieu D et al. Diffusion tensor imaging in early Alzheimer's disease. Psychiatry Res 2006; [Epub ahead of print].

54. Wallin AK, Blennow K, Andreasen N et al. CSF biomarkers for Alzheimer's disease: levels of beta-amyloid, tau, phosphorylated tau relate to clinical symptoms and survival. Dement Geriatr Cogn Disord 2006; 21(3): 131–8.

55. Tapiola T, Overmyer M, Lehtovirta M et al. The level of cerebrospinal fluid tau correlates with neurofibrillary tangles in Alzheimer's disease. NeuroReport 1997; 8: 3961–3.

56. Andreasen N. Biomarkers for Alzheimer's disease in the cerebrospinal fluid: tau, hyperphosphorylated tau and amyloid beta protein. Brain Aging 2003; 3: 7–14.

57. Parnetti L, Lanari A, Amici S et al. CSF phosphorylated tau is a possible marker for discriminating Alzheimer's disease from dementia with Lewy bodies. Neurol Sci 2001; 22: 77–8.

58. Blennow K, Hampel H. CSF markers for incipient Alzheimer's disease. Lancet Neurol 2003; 2(10): 605–13.

59. Liu T, Stern A, Roberts LJ et al. The isoprostanes: novel prostaglandin-like products of the free radical-catalyzed peroxidation of arachidonic acid. J Biomed Sci. 1999; 6(4): 226–35.

CHAPTER 4

Pathophysiology of Alzheimer's disease
Najeeb Qadi, Sina Alipour, and B Lynn Beattie

The last decade has seen unprecedented progress in the elucidation of the mechanisms and pathophysiology of Alzheimer's disease (AD). It appears increasingly clear that there is a cascade of events that act together to produce the neuropathology responsible for the disease. This chapter will review the current evidence for the contribution of a variety of mechanisms to the pathogenetic cascade of AD.

One theory of the neurobiology of AD is that it is rooted in the architectonic evolution of the human brain. The human cerebral cortex consists of three to six layers of neurons. The phylogenetically oldest part of the human cortex (archipallium) has three distinct neuronal layers and is exemplified by the hippocampus. The major part of the cortex (neocortex or neopallium), which evolves later, has six distinct cell layers and covers most of the surface of the cerebral hemispheres (see Figure 4.1).[1]

In AD, there is progressive neurodegeneration that typically follows this architectonic order, with early involvement of the hippocampus and entorhinal cortex, and later involvement of the neocortex, particularly high-order association cortices of the temporal, frontal, and parietal regions,[2] sparing the primary motor, sensory and visual cortex (unimodal cortices) until late in the disease.

HISTOPATHOLOGY

There are two main neuropathologic hallmarks in AD, the senile neuritic plaque (SP) formed around an amyloid-beta core and the neurofibrillary tangle (NFT), a paired helical filament with aggregated hyperphosphorylated tau protein (see Figure 4.2).[3] These neuropathologic lesions

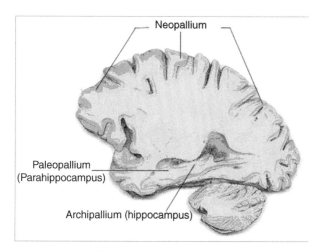

Figure 4.1 Architectonic representation of the cerebral cortex. Courtesy of Dolores Schroeder, Indiana State University, Bloomington, IN, USA, 2005, with permission.

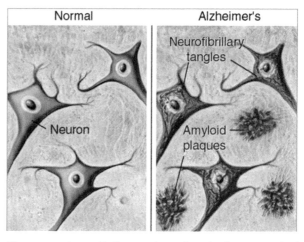

Figure 4.2 Neurofibrillary tangles and senile plaques. Medical illustration courtesy of Alzheimer's Disease Research, a program of the American Health Assistance Foundation – reproduced with permission.

likely begin to form years prior to the full clinical expression of clinical dementia, particularly within the stages of mild cognitive impairment (MCI) that are often prodromal to AD.[4]

One of the main functions of normal tau protein within neurons is to bind microtubules, promoting normal axonal transport. This binding of tau to microtubules is considered necessary to maintain the axonal integrity of neurons. There are six isoforms of tau protein in the human brain. The phosphorylation state of these tau isoforms determines their binding affinity to microtubules. In AD, tau becomes pathologically hyperphosphorylated. This triggers a cascade of events that includes tau detaching from microtubules and misfolding/aggregating into phosphorylated tau. This destabilizes microtubules, disrupts axonal transport, and leads to neuronal death.[5] NFTs are the end result of the aggregation of hyperphosphorylated tau (see Figure 4.3).[6]

NFT pathology in the brain is not unique to AD. Other conditions where NFTs occur include progressive supranuclear palsy, corticobasal degeneration, Pick's disease, Hallervorden–Spatz syndrome, Gerstmann–Straussler–Scheinker syndrome, diffuse neurofibrillary tangles with calcification, subacute sclerosing panencephalitic parkinsonism, postencephalitic parkinsonism, dementia pugilistica, Guam parkinsonism–dementia complex, and dementia with Lewy bodies.[7]

Though the molecular mechanisms that lead to this hyperphosphorylation of tau in AD are not fully understood, there is evidence that it results from an imbalance in the activity and regulation of tau kinases and phosphatases.[8] The tau kinases act to phosphorylate tau while phosphatases dephosphorylate it, providing a balance in their regulation of the phosphorylation state. An increased expression of a number of kinases has been implicated in both experimental AD models (transgenic mice) and brain tissue of AD patients (see Figure 4.4).

The upregulated kinases include glycogen synthase kinase 3 (GSK3), cyclin-dependent protein kinase 5 (CDK5), calcium/calmodulin-dependent protein kinase II (CaMK2), phospho70S6 (p70S6) kinase, mitogen activated protein (MAP) kinases ERK1/2, c-JunN terminal kinase

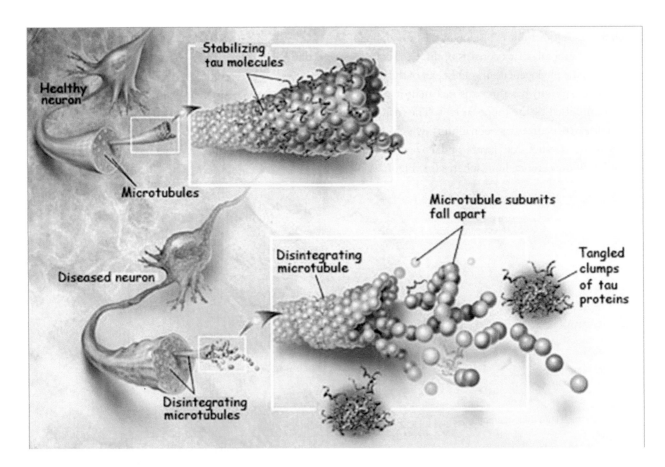

Figure 4.3 Schematic description of neurofibrillary tangle formation. Reproduced with permission from the Alzheimer's Disease Education and Referral Center, a service of the National Institute on Aging.

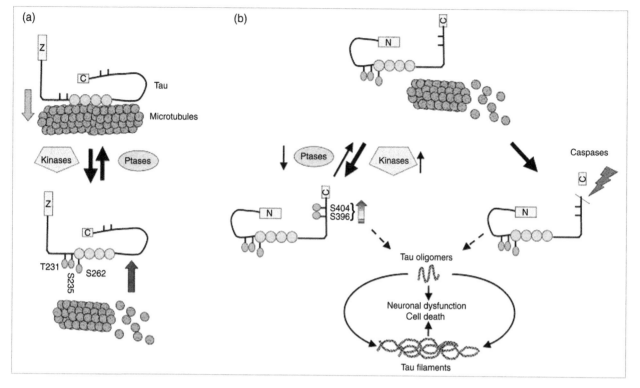

Figure 4.4 Diagram illustrating the role of tau phosphorylation in regulating tau function in a physiologic setting (a) or in a pathologic situation (b). (a) Under physiologic conditions there are balanced and dynamic changes in tau phosphorylation, which modulate tau's interactions with microtubules allowing for appropriate neuronal function. Phosphorylation at Ser262 and Thr231/Ser235 likely plays a key role in regulating tau microtubule interactions. Normal kinase and phosphatase activities keep tau–microtubule interactions tightly regulated. (b) In a pathologic state, certain toxic insults lead to a dysregulation in the balance in the activities of specific kinases and phosphatases, which results in tau being more phosphorylated at the critical microtubule regulatory sites, leading to further inappropriate phosphorylation events at fibrillogenic sites (e.g., Ser396/404) and/or cleavage by caspases at Asp421, which also increases the fibrillogenic properties of tau. These actions result in increased impairment of neuronal function. Reproduced from [8], copyright © 2004, with permission from Elsevier.

(JNK), and p38 kinase. The protein phosphatases PP1, PP2A, and PP2B have also been implicated in tau hyperphosphorylation, through their downregulation in AD.[9]

SPs can be classified into four morphologic types: diffuse, primitive, classic, and compact. It had been hypothesized previously that these different types of plaques evolve in sequence and represent stages in the life history of a single plaque type. However, recent evidence suggests that these different plaque types develop independently and, therefore, unique factors may be involved in their formation.[10] Aged individuals without AD can have some density of SPs, though most often these are diffuse and not compact as in AD.[11]

The core of SPs forms from aggregated insoluble clumps of β-amyloid polypeptides (Aβ). Aβ refers to 39–42 amino acid peptides that are formed through proteolytic cleavage of the transmembrane amyloid precursor protein (APP) (see Figure 4.5).[12]

APP isoforms range in length from 695 to 770 amino acids and are present through the membranes of a variety of organs within the human body. While the overall physiologic function of APP has not yet been determined definitely, it can serve as a cell surface receptor, as a heparin binding site, as a precursor to a growth-factor-like agent, and as a regulator of neuronal copper homeostasis.[13,14] Mice with APP knockout are 15–20% underweight compared with age-matched controls, exhibit behavioral abnormalities, and exhibit neuronal dysfunction with significant reactive astrocytosis and gliosis.[15] Whereas mice with knockout of APP and amyloid precursor-like proteins, termed APLP1 and APLP2, survive through embryonic development, but die shortly after birth. About 81% of triple mutants show cranial abnormalities and 68% triple mutants (APP, APLP1, APLP2?) have cortical dysplasia, a phenotype that resembles human type II lissencephaly.[16]

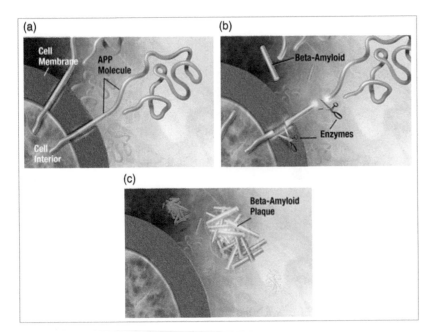

Figure 4.5 Beta-amyloid plaque formation. (a) APP is associated with the cell membrane, the thin barrier that encloses the cell. After it is made, APP sticks through the neuron's membrane, partly inside and partly outside the cell. (b) Enzymes (substances that cause or speed up a chemical reaction) act on the APP and cut it into fragments of protein; one of which is called beta-amyloid. (c) The beta amyloid fragments begin coming together into clumps outside the cell, then join other molecules and non-nerve cells to form insoluble plaques. (Reproduced with permission from the Alzheimer's Disease Education and Referral Center, a service of the National Institute on Aging.).

APP is processed through several metabolic cleavage pathways. Cleavage through α-secretase produces a soluble protein fragment (α-APP), while β- and γ-secretase cleavage forms the Aβ fragment. Aβ initially forms monofibrils, but then quickly aggregates into protofibrils that are putatively neurotoxic. They aggregate into an Aβ pleated sheet structure where amyloid becomes insoluble.[17] β-Amyloid acts to activate complement, initiates reactive changes in microglia, and stimulates the release of chemokines and cytokines. The products include the membrane attack complex, oxygen free radicals, and excess glutamate (see Figure 4.6).[18]

It has been recognized that there is microscopic evidence of a chronic inflammatory reaction in AD, where microglia and the complement cascade are activated along with T-lymphocytes.[19] Though the exact role of this inflammation in the pathogenesis of AD is still unsettled, it is generally believed that it is harmful (see Table 4.1).

Epidemiologically, there is evidence from numerous longitudinal retrospective studies and meta-analyses that the risk of AD is reduced among users of non-steroidal anti-inflammatory drugs.[20,21] These medications may reduce the inflammatory process or prevent it. Several prospective cohort studies, however, have not replicated the same findings.[22,23]

GENETICS AND AD

Familial early onset AD has been associated with mutations on chromosomes 21 (APP, Down's syndrome),[24,25]

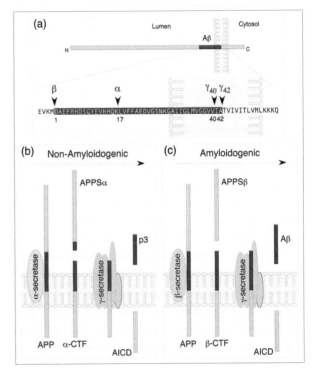

Figure 4.6 Proteolytic processing of APP. (a) Schematic structure of APP is shown with Aβ domain shaded in red and enlarged. The sites of cleavage by α, β, and γ-secretases are indicated along with Aβ numbering from the N-terminus of Aβ. (b) Non-amyloidogenic processing of APP refers to sequential processing of APP by membrane-bound α- and γ-secretases. α-Secretase cleaves within the Aβ domain, thus precluding generation of intact Aβ peptide. The fate of N-terminally truncated Aβ (p3) and APP intracellular domain (AICD) is not fully resolved. (c) Amyloidogenic processing of APP is carried out by sequential action of membrane-bound β- and γ-secretases. Reproduced form Vertivel K, Thinakaran G. Neurology 2006 66 (2) Supplement 1: S69–S73 Copyright © 2001 by AAN Enterprises, Inc.

Table 4.1 Evidence for inflammatory mechanisms in the pathogenesis of AD

Mediators	Changes	Effect
Cytokines	Increase in interleukins (IL-1, IL-6) and tumor necrosis factor expression	Increase in mediators of acute-phase reaction, generation of membrane-attack complex
Acute phase proteins	Elevation of acute-phase proteins alpha 1-antichymotrypsin, alpha 2-macroglobulin, protease inhibitors, and amyloid peptides associated with neuritic plaques	Increase in amyloid neurotoxicity, signs of inflammatory processes
Complements	Upregulation of complement system by APP	Effect on complement cascade proteins
Astrocytosis	Cytokine-induced astrocytosis	Increased production of APP
Microglia	Increase in activated microglia near AD lesions	Secretion of neurotoxins and of inflammatory cytokines, activation of HLA-DR and surface antigens, and accumulation around neuritic plaques
BBB	Disruption of BBB	

TNF = tumor necrosis factor; APP = amyloid precursor protein; BBB = blood brain barrier. Modified with permission from http://www.malattiemetaboliche.it/articoli/vol4no4c.htm#Tblone. Site visited in June 2006.

14 (presenilin 1),[26] and 1 (presenilin 2).[27] Both APP and presenilin mutations are inherited in an autosomal dominant pattern.[28] Though these autosomal dominant mutations account for <5% of all AD cases, they have informed much of our understanding of disease pathogenesis. Chromosome 21 has attracted interest for several reasons. It encodes APP and is abnormal in Down's syndrome (DS), where there are three, instead of the normal two, chromosomes. It was first recognized that DS (trisomy 21) invariably develops the neuropathology of AD by age 40[29] prior to 1991, when the first mutation of the APP gene on chromosome 21 was described.[30]

The next major genetic discovery was the elucidation of the abnormalities associated with the presenilin proteins. These proteins normally function by cutting proteins such as APP. It has been demonstrated that these complexes are closely related to γ-secretase.[31] Mutations in presenilin 1 (PS-1) and presenilin 2 (PS-2) can result in abnormal regulation of calcium in the endoplasmic reticulum,[32] leading to excessive calcium release from the endoplasmic reticulum, promoting synaptic dysfunction and neuronal death (see Figure 4.7).

Outside of the autosomal dominant mutations, there is likely an interaction between genetic and environmental factors. One genetic risk factor that has been consistently linked to AD is the apolipoprotein E (ApoE) genotype. ApoE transports cholesterol[34] and is involved in cellular repair and regeneration. It serves as a ligand for apolipoprotein receptor (LR). It also may have a role in synaptic remodeling.[35] The gene for apoE is found on chromosome 19[36] and is expressed in three different allelic forms, e2, e3, or e4. These are expressed in varying amounts in the normal individual (see Figure 4.8).

The ApoE e4 genotype is associated with an increased risk of AD.[37] Postulated mechanisms include e4 carriers having a less efficient clearance mechanism of Aβ, allowing it to build up and form SPs. The escape of tau protein from protective binding to ApoE in e4 carriers may also cause hyperphosphorylation and lead to formation of neurofibrillary tangles.[38] There is some

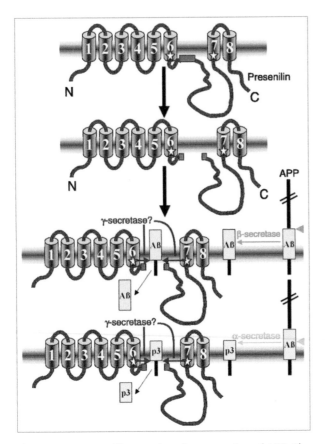

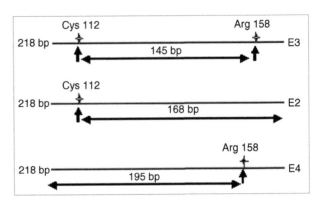

Figure 4.8 Different isoforms of ApoE (bp = base pair).

Figure 4.7 Presenilins regulate the processing of APP. The APP is a transmembrane protein that is cleaved into several Aβ peptide fragments by α-, β- or γ-secretases. Presenilin mutations that result in clinical outcomes all cause an increased production of a slightly longer (42 amino acid) variant peptide Aβ42 that is highly amyloidogenic. It has been proposed that presenilins modulate the activity of γ-secretases. Activity of the presenilins resides in their amino (N)- and carboxyl (C)-terminal fragments, which exist together with other proteins in a complex in the endoplasmic reticulum and Golgi apparatus. Reproduced with permission from [33]. Copyright © (2006) AAAS.

evidence that individuals with the e4 genotype have less efficient cholesterol transport, leading to impaired α-secretase activity (see Figure 4.9).[39]

Unlike the chromosomal mutations that are responsible for early onset AD, the presence of ApoE e4 cannot predict that the carrier will definitively develop AD. About 50% of AD is not associated with the e4 genotype.[40] Both the positive and negative predictive values of ApoE genotyping are insufficient to recommend its use as a screening test for individuals concerned about their future AD risks.

Recent research has also implicated a gene on the long arm of chromosome 10 which may be linked to AD,[41] as it acts to increase Aβ-42, a finding that still needs to be replicated.

NEUROTRANSMITTERS

There is a wide range of essential neurotransmitters that are impaired in AD. Acetylcholine has been a neurotransmitter of prominent interest since the early 1980s, when it was demonstrated that there is degeneration of cholinergic neurons in the nucleus basalis of Meynert and the basal forebrain in AD (see Figure 4.10).[42]

Other neurotransmitters, including serotonin, norepinephrine, and somatostatin, are also decreased, providing a wide range of potential relationships between the cognitive and neuropsychiatric symptoms of AD. As well, they can be identified as therapeutic targets for symptomatic treatments in AD.

CHOLESTEROL

Cholesterol is involved in the formation of the essential elements of neuronal cell membranes. It also has a vital role in the development and maintenance of neuronal plasticity and function through its effect on synapses.[43] Cholesterol influences the activity of the enzymes involved in the metabolism of the amyloid precursor protein and in the production of Aβ, though the mechanism is not fully understood.[44]. In animal studies, increased dietary cholesterol is associated with increased deposition of Aβ in the brain,[45] while in vitro studies have shown that a high cholesterol environment results in reduced production of soluble amyloid precursor protein (see Figure 4.11).[46]

ISCHEMIA

There have been a number of reported relationships between ischemic stroke events and AD. Even small,

(a)

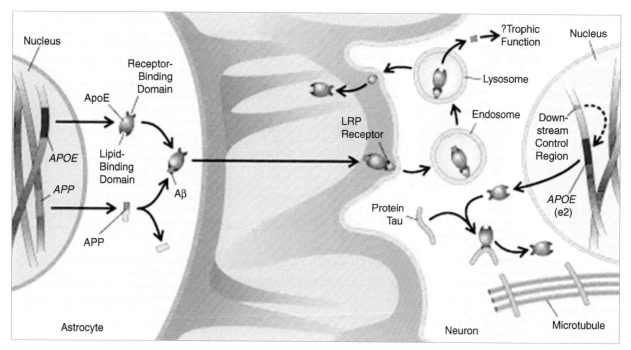

(b)

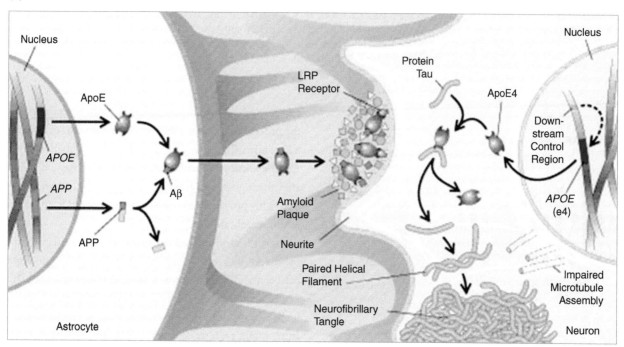

Figure 4.9 (a) Functions of ApoE. In the human brain, the protein is expressed chiefly in astrocytes (left), which also produce APP, from which the amyloid peptide Aβ is cleaved. Conceivably, ApoE conveys Aβ to brain neurons (right), where binding to LDL-related protein (LRP) might permit its internalization for a tropic function as yet unknown. In the neuronal cytoplasm, ApoE's presence may protect a binding site on tau protein. This would keep the protein available to form stabilizing cross-bridges on microtubules (www.hosppract.com/genetics/9707gen.htm) (Fig 5). Reproduced. (b) Probable role of ApoE in AD. ApoE may exit astrocytes carrying Aβ with it. Then it gets trapped by LRP on the surface of the dying neurons. Within the neuron, escape of tau protein from protective binding to ApoE may enable it to homodimerize, creating neurofibrillary tangles. In the absence of tau protein microtubules cannot assemble, which eventually leads to cell death (www.hosppract.com/genetics/9707gen.htm) (Fig 6). Reproduced.

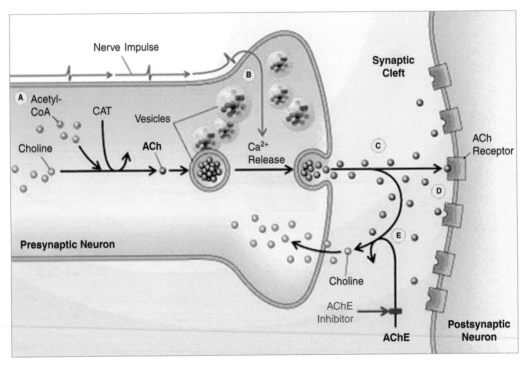

Figure 4.10 Acetylcholine (ACh) production. It is synthesized in presynaptic cholinergic neurons by choline acetyltransferase (CAT). The process entails transfer of an acetyl group to choline (A). The ACh molecules are stored in vesicles at the ends of the presynaptic neurons. Arrival of a nerve impulse triggers the release of calcium (Ca) ions, which pull the storage vesicles into position for ACh release (B). Thereafter, vesicles empty their contents into the synaptic cleft (C). Most of these molecules bind to specific receptors on adjacent postsynaptic neurons (D). Thereafter, the ACh molecules are hydrolyzed by acetylcholinesterase (AChE) (www.hosppract.com/issues/1998/11/stahl.htm). Reproduced.

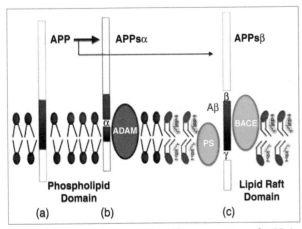

Figure 4.11 Putative model of the processing of APP in relation to the lipid composition of membranes. (a) APP is a transmembrane protein. (b) Cleavage of APP by α-secretases, such as ADAM10, produces APPsα, which requires a membrane domain that is cholesterol poor, such as phospholipid domains. (c) Cleavage of APP by the β- and γ-secretases, BACE, and presenilin (PS) produces Aβ and APPsβ. This step requires a membrane domain that is cholesterol rich, such as a lipid raft. APP processing can be directed toward α-secretase or β/γ-secretase pathways by modulating the cholesterol content of the membranes. Lipid identities: blue, phospholipid; green, sphingolipids; yellow, cholesterol. Reproduced from [47] with permission.

scarce, and asymptomatic cerebral infarcts can increase the probability of expressing clinical symptoms of dementia in individuals with existing SP and NFT pathology.[48] Another link to vascular changes in AD may be mediated through cerebral amyloid angiopathy (CAA). This is a highly prevalent disorder in AD where Aβ is deposited within cerebral blood vessel walls.[49]

Several randomized clinical trials and observational cohort studies have demonstrated that there are links between midlife hypertension and AD (see Figure 4.12).[50] Dysregulated cerebral blood flow and hypoperfusion of brain regions due to arteriosclerosis of the cerebral vasculature might precede dementia symptoms by many years.[51] It has also been shown that the association between atherosclerosis and dementia is particularly strong in those with the ApoE e4 genotype.[52]

CONCLUSION

Much of the elucidation of the pathophysiology of AD has revolved around the pathologic findings of SPs and

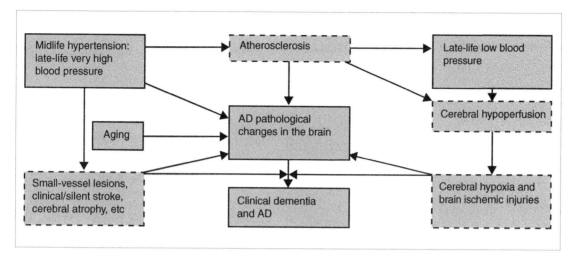

Figure 4.12 Possible biological pathways that link midlife hypertension and late-life low blood pressure to AD and dementia. Boxes with solid lines include risk factors. Boxes with dashed lines represent possible pathophysiologic pathways linking these factors to AD pathologic changes and clinical expression of dementia. Reproduced from [50] with permission.

NFTs. The key constituents of Aβ-42 and hyperphosphorylated tau have a vital role in the pathogenic sequence with some emerging elucidation of their interrelationship. Downstream to the deposition of SPs and NFTs there is both resulting inflammation and oxidative stress that add to this pathologic cascade. There is a resultant loss of neurotransmission and neurotransmitter function. The significance of vascular injury is recognized to have particular importance as it interacts with other parts of the pathologic cascade. With this progress in understanding the pathogenesis of AD, treatment targets are better defined to more definitively treat this neurodegenerative disease.

REFERENCES

1. Mesulum MM. Principles of Behavioural Neurology. Philadelphia: FA Davis Company, 1985.

2. Price JL, Ko AI, Wade MJ et al. Neuron number in the entorhinal cortex and CA1 in preclinical Alzheimer disease. Arch Neurol 2001; 58(9): 1395–402.

3. Khachaturian ZS. Diagnosis of Alzheimer's disease. Arch Neurol 1985; 2(11): 1097–105.

4. Guillozet AL, Weintraub S, Mash DC et al. Neurofibrillary tangles, amyloid, and memory in aging and mild cognitive impairment. Arch Neurol 2003; 60(5): 729–36.

5. Trojanowski JQ, Schmidt ML, Otvos L Jr et al. Vulnerability of the neuronal cytoskeleton in aging and Alzheimer disease: widespread involvement of all three major filament systems. Annu Rev Gerontol Geriatr 1990; 10: 167–82.

6. Kosik KS. Tau protein and Alzheimer's disease. Curr Opin Cell Biol 1990; 2(1): 101–4.

7. Lee VM, Goedert M, Trojanowski JQ. Neurodegenerative tauopathies. Annu Rev Neurosci 2001; 24: 1121–59.

8. Stoothoff WH, Johnson GV. Tau phosphorylation: physiological and pathological consequences. Biochim Biophys Acta 2005; 1739(2–3): 280–97.

9. Iqbal K, Alonso Adel C, Chen S et al. Tau pathology in Alzheimer disease and other tauopathies. Biochim Biophys Acta 2005; 1739(2–3): 198–210.

10. Armstrong RA. Beta-amyloid plaques: stages in life history or independent origin? Dement Geriatr Cogn Disord 1998; 9(4): 227–38.

11. Dickson DW. Neuropathological diagnosis of Alzheimer's disease: a perspective from longitudinal clinicopathological studies. Neurobiol Aging 1997; 18(4 Suppl): S21–6.

12. Sahasrabudhe SR, Brown AM, Hulmes JD et al. Enzymatic generation of the amino terminus of the beta-amyloid peptide. J Biol Chem 1993; 268(22): 16699–705.

13. Fiore F, Zambrano N, Minopoli G et al. The regions of the Fe65 protein homologous to the phosphotyrosine interaction/phosphotyrosine binding domain of Shc bind the intracellular domain of the Alzheimer's amyloid precursor protein. J Biol Chem 1995; 270, 30 853–6.

14. Maynard CJ, Cappai R, Volitakis I et al. Overexpression of Alzheimer's disease amyloid-beta opposes the age-dependent elevations of brain copper and iron. J Biol Chem 2002; 277(47): 44670–6.

15. Zheng H, Jiang M, Trumbauer ME et al. Beta-Amyloid precursor protein-deficient mice show reactive gliosis and decreased locomotor activity. Cell 1995; 81(4): 525–31.

16. Herms J, Anliker B, Heber S et al. Cortical dysplasia resembling human type 2 lissencephaly in mice lacking all three APP family members. EMBO J 2004; 23(20): 4106–15.

17. Hilbich C, Kisters-Woike B, Reed J et al. Aggregation and secondary structure of synthetic amyloid beta A4 peptides of Alzheimer's disease. J Mol Biol 1991; 218(1): 149–63.

18. McGeer EG, McGeer PL. The importance of inflammatory mechanisms in Alzheimer disease. Exp Gerontol 1998; 33(5): 371–8.

19. Aisen PS. Inflammation and Alzheimer disease. Mol Chem Neuropathol 1996; 28(1–3): 83–8.

20. in't Veld BA, Launer LJ, Hoes AW et al. NSAIDs and incident Alzheimer's disease. The Rotterdam Study. Neurobiol Aging 1998; 19: 607–11.

21. McGeer PL, Schulzer M, McGeer EG. Arthritis and anti-inflammatory agents as possible protective factors for Alzheimer's disease: a review of 17 epidemiologic studies. Neurology 1996; 47: 425–32.

22. Aisen PS, Schafer KA, Grundman M et al. Effects of rofecoxib or naproxen versus placebo on Alzheimer's disease progression: a randomized controlled trial. JAMA 2003; 289: 2819–26.

23. Reines SA, BlockNessly ML, Lines CR et al. Rofecoxib Protocol 091 Study Group. Rofecoxib: no effect on Alzheimer's disease in a 1-year, randomized, blinded, controlled study. Neurology 2004; 62: 66–71.

24. Axelman K, Basun H, Winblad B et al. A large Swedish family with Alzheimer's disease with a codon 670/671 amyloid precursor protein mutation. A clinical and genealogical investigation. Arch Neurol 1994; 51(12): 1193–7.

25. Brugge KL, Nichols SL, Salmon DP et al. Cognitive impairment in adults with Down's syndrome: similarities to early cognitive changes in Alzheimer's disease. Neurology 1994; 44(2): 232–8.

26. Kennedy AM, Newman SK, Frackowiak RS et al. Chromosome 14 linked familial Alzheimer's disease. A clinico-pathological study of a single pedigree. Brain 1995; 118(Pt 1): 185–205.

27. Levy-Lahad E, Wijsman EM, Nemens E et al. A familial Alzheimer's disease locus on chromosome 1. Science 1995; 269(5226): 970–3.

28. van Duijn CM, Hendriks L, Farrer LA et al. A population-based study of familial Alzheimer disease: linkage to chromosomes 14, 19, and 21. Am J Hum Genet 1994; 55(4): 714–27.

29. Wisniewski KE, Dalton AJ, McLachlan C et al. Alzheimer's disease in Down's syndrome: clinicopathologic studies. Neurology 1985; 35(7): 957–61.

30. Goate A, Chartier-Harlin MC, Mullan M et al. Segregation of a missense mutation in the amyloid precursor protein gene with familial Alzheimer's disease. Nature 1991; 349(6311): 704–6.

31. Brunkan AL, Goate AM. Presenilin function and gamma-secretase activity. J Neurochem 2005; 93(4): 769–92.

32. Leissring MA, LaFerla FM, Callamaras N et al. Subcellular mechanisms of presenilin-mediated enhancement of calcium signaling. Neurobiol Dis 2001; 8(3): 469–78.

33. Haass C, De Strooper B. The presenilins in Alzheimer's disease – proteolysis holds the key. Science 1999; 29: 916–19.

34. Poirier J. Apolipoprotein E and cholesterol metabolism in the pathogenesis and treatment of Alzheimer's disease. Trends Mol Med 2003; 9: 94–101.

35. Mahley RW, Nathan BP, Pitas RE. Apolipoprotein E. Structure, function, and possible roles in Alzheimer's disease. Ann NY Acad Sci 1996; 777: 139–45.

36. Olaisen B, Teisberg P, Gedde-Dahl T Jr. The locus for apolipoprotein E (apoE) is linked to the complement component C3 (C3) locus on chromosome 19 in man. Hum Genet 1982; 62(3): 233–6.

37. Corder EH, Saunders AM, Strittmatter WJ et al. Gene dose of apolipoprotein E type 4 allele and the risk of Alzheimer's disease in late onset families. Science 1993; 261(5123): 921–3.

38. Tesseur I, Van Dorpe J, Spittaels K et al. Expression of human apolipoprotein E4 in neurons causes hyperphosphorylation of protein tau in the brains of transgenic mice. Am J Pathol 2000; 156(3): 951–64.

39. Dupuy AM, Mas E, Ritchie K, Descomps B et al. The relationship between apolipoprotein E4 and lipid metabolism is impaired in Alzheimer's disease. Gerontology 2001; 47(4): 213–18.

40. Myers AJ, Goate AM. The genetics of late-onset Alzheimer's disease. Curr Opin Neurol 2001; 14(4): 433–40.

41. Bertram L, Blacker D, Mullin K et al. Evidence for genetic linkage of Alzheimer's disease to chromosome 10q. Science 2000; 290(5500): 2302–3.

42. Whitehouse PJ, Price DL, Clark AW et al. Alzheimer disease: evidence for selective loss of cholinergic neurons in the nucleus basalis. Ann Neurol 1981; 10(2): 122–6.

43. Pfrieger FW. Cholesterol homeostasis and function in neurons of the central nervous system. Cell Mol Life Sci 2003; 60: 1158–71.

44. Shobab LA, Hsiung G-YR, Feldman HH. Cholesterol in Alzheimer's disease. Lancet Neurol 2005; 4: 841–52.

45. Shie FS, Jin LW, Cook DG et al. Diet-induced hypercholesterolemia enhances brain A beta accumulation in transgenic mice. Neuroreport 2002; 13: 455–9.

46. Racchi M, Baetta R, Salvietti N et al. Secretory processing of amyloid precursor protein is inhibited by increase in cellular cholesterol content. Biochem J 1997; 322: 893–8.

47. Wolozin B. A fluid connection: cholesterol and Abeta. Proc Natl Acad Sci USA 2001; 98(10): 5371–3.

48. Pasquier F, Leys D. Why are stroke patients prone to develop dementia? J Neurol 1997; 244(3): 135–42.

49. Weller RO, Massey A, Newman TA et al. Cerebral amyloid angiopathy: amyloid beta accumulates in putative interstitial fluid drainage pathways in Alzheimer's disease. Am J Pathol 1998; 153(3): 725–33.

50. Qiu C, Winblad B, Fratiglioni L. The age-dependent relation of blood pressure to cognitive function and dementia. Lancet Neurol 2005; 4(8): 487–99.

51. Jellinger KA. Alzheimer disease and cerebrovascular pathology: an update. J Neural Transm 2002; 109(5–6): 813–36.

52. Hofman A, Ott A, Breteler MMB et al. Atherosclerosis, apolipoprotein E, and prevalence of dementia and Alzheimer's disease in the Rotterdam Study. Lancet 1997; 349: 151–4.

CHAPTER 5

Neuropathology of Alzheimer's disease
Ian RA Mackenzie

INTRODUCTION

In 1907, Alois Alzheimer described changes in the brain of a 56-year-old woman, dying of progressive dementia.[1] Using a newly developed histologic staining technique (the Bielschowsky silver impregnation method) Alzheimer demonstrated the presence of neurofibrillary tangles and 'miliary foci' (senile plaques) in the post-mortem brain tissue. Although others had described these microscopic changes previously, it was Alzheimer who first drew attention to their relationship with clinical dementia. Despite the many significant advances that have recently been made in our understanding of the clinical, biochemical, and genetic aspects of Alzheimer's disease (AD), definitive diagnosis is still dependent on the identification of these same pathologic changes in brain tissue.

GROSS PATHOLOGY

The brain is usually atrophic, often weighing less than 1000 g, with the degree of tissue loss roughly correlating with the severity of cognitive decline. Cerebral atrophy tends to be diffuse, affecting the frontal, temporal, and parietal lobes with particular involvement of the mesial temporal structures (hippocampus and parahippocampal gyrus) (Figure 5.1). The occipital lobes and primary motor and sensory cortex are generally spared. Tissue loss is manifest by narrowing of the cerebral gyri, widening of sulci, thinning of the cortical ribbon, and enlargement of the ventricles, especially the temporal horn. In some cases, there is decreased pigmentation of the substantia nigra, however this is mild unless there is coexisting Lewy body disease. Lesions of cerebrovascular

disease may coexist and their presence does not exclude the diagnosis of AD.

MICROSCOPIC PATHOLOGY

There are no specific changes outside the brain. Affected areas show a variety of non-specific degenerative changes including neuronal loss, reactive gliosis, and microglial activation. The degree of neuronal loss varies and may reach 60% in the hippocampal pyramidal layer and >80% in the nucleus basalis and some regions of the frontal and temporal neocortex. Synaptic reduction can be demonstrated by electron microscopy and reduced immunoreactivity for various synaptic proteins.

The pathologic changes that are considered to be most characteristic of AD are the presence of numerous senile plaques and neurofibrillary tangles in the cerebral neocortex (Figure 5.2). Although these changes can be seen with routine hematoxylin and eosin stain (HE), they are much better demonstrated with various special histochemical stains and immunohistochemistry.

Senile plaques (SPs) are spherical lesions, measuring up to 200 μm in diameter. They consist of a focal deposit of extracellular amyloid, associated with various localized cellular changes. The protein that deposits as amyloid in the AD brain is Aβ (also known as β peptide, A4 peptide, βA4, amyloid β protein), a ~4 kDa peptide that ranges in length from 39 to 43 amino acids, due to variability in the C-terminus. Most of the Aβ that accumulates in SP is the longer A$\beta_{42,43}$ species, while Aβ_{40} predominates in amyloid angiopathy (see below). Aβ is produced through the proteolytic cleavage of a normal transmembrane protein, the amyloid precursor protein

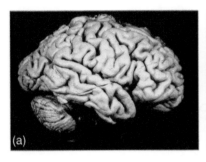
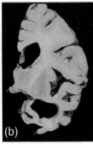

Figure 5.1 Gross appearance of a post-mortem brain with Alzheimer's disease. (a) Moderate, diffuse cerebral atrophy with narrowing of gyri and widening of sulci. (b) Coronal hemisection at level of basal ganglia, showing ventricular dilatation and atrophy of the hippocampus.

(a)

(b)

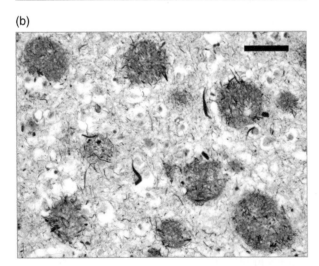

Figure 5.2 Alzheimer's disease is characterized by numerous senile plaques and neurofibrillary tangles in the cerebral neocortex. Bielschowsky silver stain, scale bar: (a) 500 μm, (b) 100 μm.

(APP). APP is widely expressed by a variety of cell types, including neurons. Usually, APP is cleaved in the middle of the Aβ sequence; however, an alternate processing pathway exists that results in the production of the intact Aβ fragment (Figure 5.3).

What is amyloid? The term amyloid refers to any amorphous, eosinophilic, extracellular protein deposit that has specific staining characteristics, such as binding Congo red stain and showing birefringence with polarized light. All amyloid is composed of 8 to 10 nm diameter protein fibrils that aggregate to form a 'cross-β' pleated sheet configuration. Although a number of biochemically diverse proteins can form amyloid, it is this highly regular three-dimensional physical structure that imparts the characteristic staining pattern.

Several different morphologic types of SP are recognized (Figure 5.4). In *neuritic* SPs, the focal deposit of fibrillar amyloid contains a cluster of radially oriented, abnormally distended neuronal processes. These 'dystrophic neurites' are terminal dendrites and axons that contain dense bodies and vesicular structures, sometimes mixed with paired helical filaments (see below). In *classical* neuritic SPs, the dystrophic neurites surround a central dense amyloid core, with less compact amyloid fibrils deposited between the neurites (Figure 5.4a). *Primitive* neuritic SPs lack a well-defined central core of amyloid (Figure 5.4b). *Burned-out* plaques have only a dense amyloid core, in the absence of any cellular component (Figure 5.4c). Finally, *diffuse* SPs are a focal

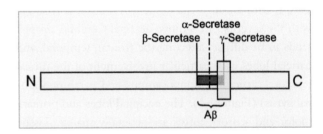

Figure 5.3 Diagramatic representation of the amyloid precursor protein (APP) (yellow) inserted in the cell membrane (pale blue). Most often, enzymatic processing involves α-secretase cleavage in the middle of the Aβ region (red). However, there is an alternate pathway in which β- and γ-secretase activity results in production of the amyloidogenic Aβ peptide.

amorphous deposit of non-fibrillar Aβ (pre-amyloid) that is not associated with any alteration in the cellular neuropil (therefore, they are not 'neuritic') (Figure 5.4d). Different staining techniques and immunohistochemistry can be used to demonstrate each of the components and distinguish the different SP subtypes (Figure 5.5). Although it is suspected that the different types of SP represent a continuum, with one type maturing or evolving into the next (diffuse to primitive, to classical, to burned out), this is difficult to prove.

In addition to amyloid, a variety of other molecules may be present in the extracellular component of SP, including immune system proteins (such as complement and cytokines), growth factors, adhesion molecules, ApoE, and proteoglycans, to name a few. Neuritic SPs are also associated with a localized glial cell reaction;

activated microglia are often present within the plaque boundary and reactive astrocytes are found in the adjacent neuropil (Figure 5.6).

It is the presence of frequent neuritic SPs in the neocortex that is most characteristic of AD. Diffuse SPs tend to be numerous in AD as well, but because they are also a common finding in the brains of non-demented elderly individuals, they are not disease-specific (see below). The anatomic distribution of SP in AD is widespread and does not show the degree of topographic hierarchy seen with neurofibrillary degeneration. None-the-less, higher order association cortex tends to have the highest density of SPs, and primary motor and sensory cortex the least (Figure 5.7).[2] The hippocampus often has relatively few plaques. There may be numerous SPs in the striatum and cerebellar

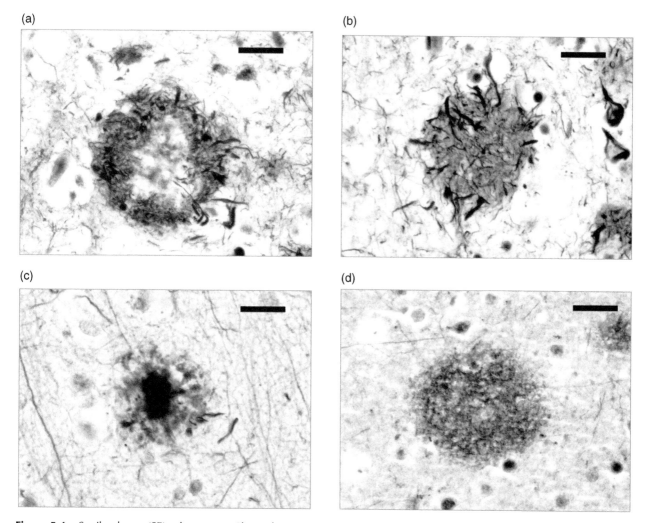

Figure 5.4 Senile plaque (SP) subtypes. (a) *Classical neuritic SP* with a central amyloid core surrounded by a ring of dystrophic neurites. (b) *Primitive neuritic plaque* with focal collection of neurites but no compact amyloid core. (c) *Burned-out plaque* with amyloid core but few associated neurites. (d) Diffuse SP consisting of a focal deposit of non-fibrillar Aβ peptide. Bielschowsky silver stain, scale bar: (a–d) 50 μm.

(a)

(b)

(c)

(d)

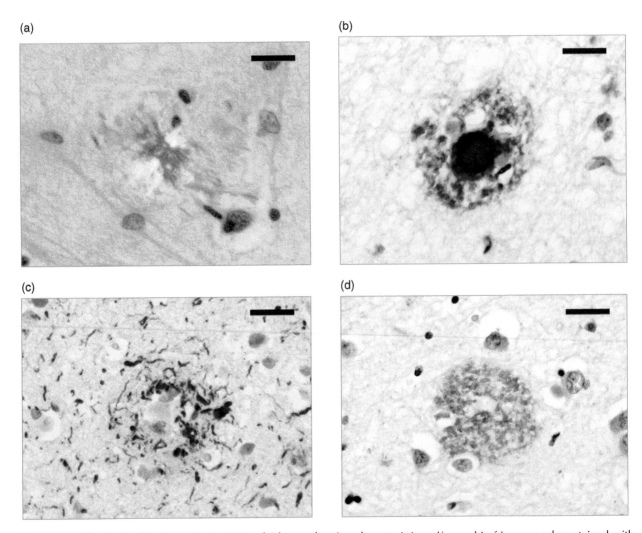

Figure 5.5 Classical senile plaque (a–c). (a) Amyloid core showing characteristic red/green birefringence when stained with Congo red and viewed using polarized light. (b) Aβ immunohistochemistry demonstrates central compact amyloid core and more dispersed amyloid at periphery. (c) Dystrophic neurites are immunoreactive for hyperphosphorylated tau. (d) Diffuse senile plaque immunostained for Aβ peptide. Scale bar: (a–d) 50 μm.

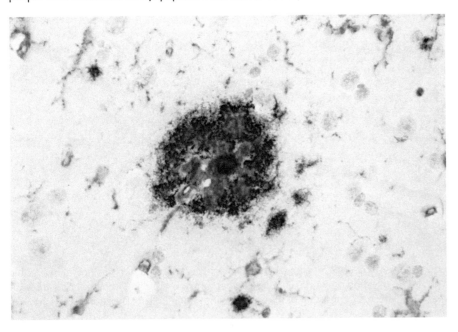

Figure 5.6 Activated microglia, expressing major histocompatibility complex type II (MHC II) (brown), infiltrating a classical senile plaque (immunostained for Aβ, black). There are also increased numbers of activated microglia in surrounding neuropil. Scale bar: 50 μm.

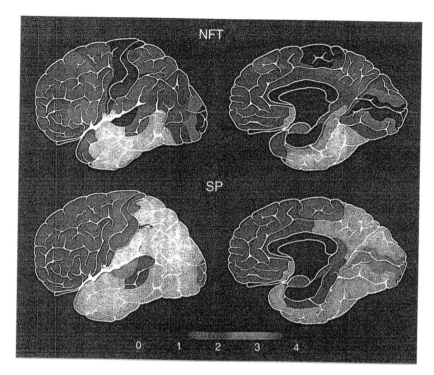

Figure 5.7 Regional distribution of neurofibrillary tangles (NFT) and senile plaques (SP) in Alzheimer's disease. Reproduced with permission from Arnold et al. The topographical and neuroanatomical distribution of neurofibrillary tangles and neuritic plaques in the cerebral cortex of patients with Alzheimer's disease. Cereb Cortex 1991; 1: 103–16.[2]

molecular layer, however these are almost exclusively of the diffuse type.

Neurofibrillary tangles (NFTs) are intracellular collections of abnormal filaments that displace the normal cytoplasmic organelles. In pyramidal neurons, such as in the hippocampus, NFTs tend to fill much of the cell body and apical dendrite, giving a characteristic 'flame' shape (Figure 5.8a, b). In neurons with a more rounded contour, such as the nucleus basalis, the NFTs are more globose. In some anatomic locations, such as the hippocampus, extracellular (ghost) tangles may persist in the extracellular space after the neuron dies (Figure 5.8c).

The filaments that compose NFTs have a characteristic ultrastructure, consisting of two ribbon-like strands, twisted around one another to form a helix ('paired-helical filaments', PHFs). The diameter of each PHF alternates between 20 nm and 8 nm with a regular periodicity of 80 nm (Figure 5.9).[3] The major protein component of PHF is the microtubule associated protein tau, that is in an abnormally hyperphosphorylated form (Figure 5.8d).

In AD, NFTs tend to be most numerous in the limbic structures of the mesial temporal lobe, including the hippocampus, sibiculum, amygdala, and entorhinal and transentorhinal cortex. The neocortex is involved in a hierarchical fashion, with the higher-order association cortex more affected than the unimodal association cortex, and the primary sensory and motor cortex are relatively spared. NFTs are frequently present in certain subcortical nuclei such as the nucleus basalis, limbic nuclei of the thalamus, amygdala, locus ceruleus, substantia nigra, and raphe nuclei of the brainstem.

NFTs are also a frequent finding in non-demented elderly individuals, especially in the mesial temporal lobe. Braak and Braak have shown that neurofibrillary pathology in the brain accumulates in a hierarchical topographic fashion, with the transentorhinal cortex affected first (stages I and II), followed by the entorhinal cortex and hippocampus (stages III and IV), and finally the isocortex (stages V and VI) (Figure 5.10).[4,5] Most patients with dementia are found to have stage V or VI pathology, while those at lower stages are usually not demented.

Neuropil threads are another form of neurofibrillary degeneration in which PHF accumulates in distal dendrites and axons. These short thread-like structures have the same staining characteristics as NFTs and are widely distributed throughout the gray matter in AD (Figure 5.8d). As mentioned above, some of the dystrophic neurites of senile plaques also contain PHFs.

OTHER MICROSCOPIC CHANGES

Cerebral amyloid angiopathy (CAA) refers to the deposition of amyloid in the walls of blood vessels of the brain (Figure 5.11). In AD, the protein that accumulates as

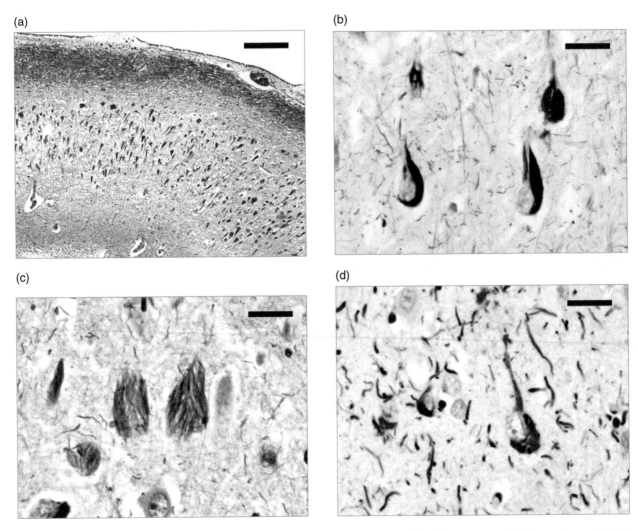

Figure 5.8 Neurofibrillary tangles (NFTs). (a) Numerous NFTs in CA2 region of the hippocampus. (b) Flame-shaped NFTs in pyramidal neurons of hippocampus. (c) Ghost tangles remain after affected neuron has degenerated. (d) NFTs and neuropil threads contain abnormal tau protein. (a–c) Bielschowsky silver stain, (d) immunohistochemistry for hyperphosphorylated tau protein. Scale bar: (a) 500 μm, (b–d) 50 μm.

amyloid in vessel walls is also Aβ, although the shorter Aβ$_{40}$ peptide predominates. CAA primarily affects small arteries and arterioles of the leptomeninges and penetrating vessels of cerebral and cerebellar cortex. Capillaries and veins may also be involved, however vessels of the white matter and deep gray nuclei are generally spared. The pattern of amyloid deposition in a particular vessel may be patchy and focal or contiguous and circumferential. CAA may produce a number of morphologic changes in the affected vessels including stenosis or occlusion, aneurysmal dilatation, or vessel-within-vessel (double-barrel) formation. Rarely, CAA is associated with a giant cell vasculitis. Complications include both ischemic injury and spontaneous lobar cerebral hemorrhage. CAA is a common, but not inevitable, feature in AD (found in >80% of cases) and is also found in some

elderly non-demented individuals. In AD, the severity and distribution of CAA does not seem to correlate with that of SP. The source of the Aβ that deposits in cerebral blood vessels is uncertain, with possible origins being (1) systemic tissues, reaching the brain in the circulating blood, (2) neuronal release into brain interstitial fluid, or (3) local production by the cellular component of the vessel wall.

Granulovacuolar degeneration (GVD) mainly involves hippocampal CA1 and CA2 pyramidal neurons (Figure 5.12a). Affected cells have multiple small intracytoplasmic vacuoles, each containing one or more central granules. The granules are basophilic, argyrophilic, and immunoreactive for various cytoskeletal proteins and ubiquitin. These structures are thought to be derived from autophagic lysosomes.

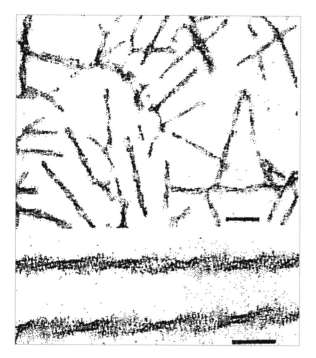

Figure 5.9 Ultrastructure of paired helical filaments (PHFs) extracted from AD brain. Reprinted with permission from Lee et al. A68: a major subunit of paired helical filaments and derivatized forms of normal tau. Science 1991; 256: 675–8.[3] Copyright 1991 AAAS.

Hirano bodies are eosinophilic rod-like structures, found mainly in the CA1 sector of the hippocampus (Figure 5.12b). Although they often appear to be immediately adjacent to the neuronal cell body, they are actually intracellular, within neuronal processes. They have a highly-organized, paracrystalline ultrastructure and are immunoreactive for a variety of cytoskeletal proteins including actin, neurofilament, and microtubule associated proteins. Hirano bodies are often numerous in AD but are also common in other neurodegenerative conditions and normal aging.

Chronic inflammation is a consistent feature of the AD brain. As mentioned above, activated, immune competent microglial cells are commonly present in SP and are increased in numbers throughout the brain (Figure 5.6). Levels of various immune system proteins are also elevated in AD brain tissue. Although some of this may be a non-specific response to neurodegeneration, there is mounting evidence that inflammatory mechanisms play an important role in the pathogenesis of AD.[6]

AD VERSUS AGE-RELATED PATHOLOGY

Although SPs and NFTs are considered to be the characteristic pathologic changes of AD, they are not specific.

Autopsy examination of non-demented individuals discloses at least some plaques and tangles in the majority, over the age of 60 years. Although the number and distribution of SPs may approach that seen in AD, most of the SPs in neurologically normal elderly patients are of the early 'diffuse' type, with neuritic plaques being uncommon (Figure 5.13). Neurofibrillary pathology is also increasingly common with advancing age but tends to have a more restricted anatomic distribution, being limited to the limbic structures of the mesial temporal lobe. It is not clear what proportion of these cases represents preclinical AD versus a limited age-related change that would not have progressed.

PATHOLOGIC DIAGNOSTIC CRITERIA FOR AD

Since there is no absolute qualitative difference that distinguishes the brains of demented patients from those of non-demented elderly individuals, the pathologic diagnosis of AD depends on identifying quantitative differences. Establishing such criteria is difficult, due to the degree of overlap in the pathology of the two groups (which may indicate that individuals have different thresholds) and variation in the sensitivity of the staining techniques used in different labs. As indicated in Table 5.1, the diagnostic criteria for AD have evolved over the past few decades and will likely continue to do so.[4,7–9]

PATHOLOGY OF FAMILIAL AD

In general, the pathologic changes seen in both early- and late-onset familial AD tend to be similar to those seen in sporadic cases. Inheritance of the apoE ε4 allele and some mutations in the APP and presenilin genes tend to be associated with more abundant amyloid deposition, either in the form of SPs or CAA. Some PS-1 mutations are found to have an unusual type of amyloid deposit, referred to as 'cotton-wool' plaques (Figure 5.14).

AD COMBINED WITH OTHER PATHOLOGY ('MIXED DEMENTIA')

Post-mortem neuropathologic examination of demented individuals frequently demonstrates AD in combination

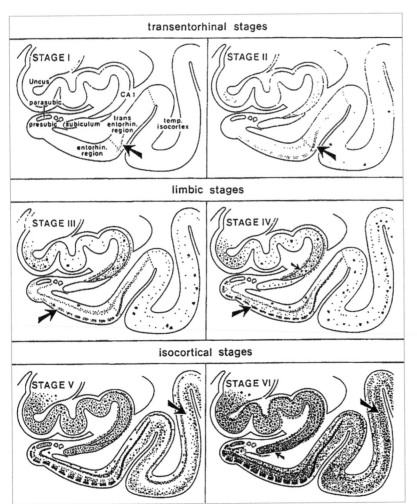

Figure 5.10 Progessive accumulation of neurofibrillary pathology, as proposed by Braak and Braak. Neurofibrillary tangles (NFTs) first appear in the transentorhinal region (stages I and II), followed by the entorhinal cortex and hippocampus (stages III and IV), and finally the neocortex (stages V and VI). Reproduced from Braak H, Braak E. Evolution of the neuropathology of Alzheimer's disease. Acta Neurol Scand 1996; 165(Suppl): 3–12,[5] with the permission of Blackwell Publishing.

with other pathologic changes that could potentially have contributed to dementia. The most common co-existing conditions are cerebrovascular disease (CVD), Lewy body disease (LBD), or both. The frequency of these cases of 'mixed dementia' is difficult to determine, due to a lack of consensus as to what constitutes a *significant* degree of other pathology. However, some studies have shown that close to 50% of AD cases have one or more additional pathologic processes.[10] Reasons for the high frequency of CVD in AD include (1) chance coexistence of common conditions, (2) shared risk factors (i.e. ApoE genotype), and (3) synergistic physiologic processes (i.e. chronic ischemia increases amyloid production and, conversely, neurons are more susceptible to oxidative stress in the presence of elevated Aβ amyloid). The basis for the coexistence of AD and LBD is less clear, however there is growing evidence that the biochemical processes involved in these diseases (aberrant metabolism of tau and α-synuclein, respectively) may be closely linked. A number of

clinicopathologic correlative studies have supported the hypothesis that when other pathologies occur in AD, they may contribute to the severity and/or progression of dementia.[11]

PATHOGENESIS OF AD

Although both SPs and NFTs are generally considered to be characteristic of AD, controversy remains as to the relationship between these lesions and which process, if either, is central to disease pathogenesis. Studies showing that the numbers of NFTs correlate better with the degree of dementia are interpreted by some as indicating that neurofibrillary degeneration is the more important process. Against this view, however, is the fact that NFTs are also a common feature in a wide range of other neurodegenerative conditions. The common finding of SPs in non-demented elderly individuals and the relatively poor correlation between amyloid burden

(a)

(b)

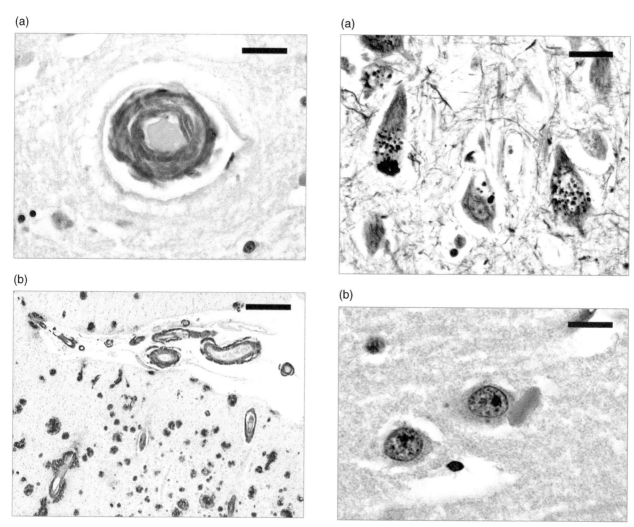

Figure 5.11 Cerebral amyloid angiopathy. Amyloid accumulation in the walls of small and medium sized blood vessels in the cerebral cortex and leptomeninges. (a) Congo red stain, (b) Aβ immunohistochemistry. Scale bar: (a) 50 μm, (b) 500 μm.

Figure 5.12 (a) Granulovacuolar degeneration of multiple pyramidal neurons in CA2 region of hippocampus. Bielschowsky silver stain. (b) Eosinophilic Hirano body adjacent to a CA1 hippocampal neuron. Hematoxylin and eosin. Scale bar: (a, b) 50 μm.

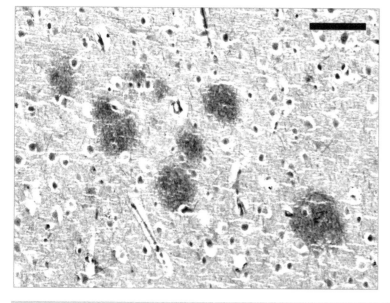

Figure 5.13 Numerous diffuse senile plaques in the post-mortem brain of a non-demented aged individual. Bielschowsky silver stain, scale bar: 100 μm.

Table 5.1 Neuropathologic diagnostic criteria for Alzheimer's disease

Criteria	Method	Issues
Khachaturian (1985)[7]	• Based on minimum number of SPs per mm^2 • Required number of SPs increases with advancing age	• Does not distinguish between SP types • Does not require history of dementia • Many non-demented elderly with diffuse SPs fulfill criteria for AD
CERAD (1991)[8]	• Semiquantitative assessment of neuritic SPs • SP frequency combined with patient age to generate an age-related plaque score • Age-related plaque score integrated with clinical information regarding the presence or absence of dementia to determine level of certainty of diagnosis	• Presence of NFTs not required • Cases with numerous SPs but few NFTs considered AD (including many cases of dementia with Lewy bodies)
Braak (1991)[4]	• Based on topographic staging of NFT • Higher stages with NFTs in neocortex (stages V, VI) consistent with AD	• SP not evaluated • Some cases don't fit into defined stages
NIA/Reagan Institute (1997)[9]	• Semiquantitative evaluation of SPs (as per CERAD) • Topographic staging of NFTs (as per Braak) • Determine likelihood that AD is the cause of dementia (high if frequent SPs and Braak stage V/VI, intermediate if moderate SPs and Braak stage III/IV, low if sparse SPs and Braak stage I/II)	• Uncertain how to interpret cases in which the frequency of SPs and NFTs do not correlate (i.e. frequent SPs, Braak stage I/II)

SP, senile plaque; NFT, neurofibrillary tangle; CERAD, consortium to establish a registry for Alzheimer's disease; NIA, National Institute on Aging.

and dementia have prompted some to dismiss SP formation as being an unimportant secondary phenomenon in AD. However, over the past few decades, support has grown for the 'amyloid cascade' hypothesis of AD, in which the accumulation of Aβ amyloid in brain tissue is believed to be an early and necessary step, that then triggers a series of events (including neurofibrillary degeneration) that lead to neurodegeneration and

dementia. Some of the evidence to support the central role of Aβ in AD pathogenesis includes (1) evidence for Aβ neurotoxicity, (2) cross-sectional studies of patient populations known to develop AD, showing Aβ accumulation to be the earliest recognizable change, and (3) the fact that all the genetic factors that cause or increase the risk of AD affect the production or clearance of Aβ amyloid.[12] Further clarification of the sequence of

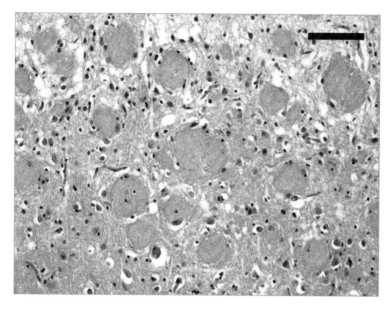

Figure 5.14 'Cotton-wool' plaques with no amyloid core and minimal neuritic pathology in a patient with familial Alzheimer's disease caused by a mutation in the presenilin-1 gene. Hematoxylin and eosin, scale bar: 100 µm.

pathologic events that cause AD dementia will be a crucial step in developing logical and effective treatment strategies.

REFERENCES

1. Alzheimer A. Ueber eine eigenartige Erkrankung der Hirnrinde. Allg Z Psychiatr 1907; 64: 146–8.

2. Arnold SE, Hyman BT, Flory J et al. The topographical and neuroanatomical distribution of neurofibrillary tangles and neuritic plaques in the cerebral cortex of patients with Alzheimer's disease. Cereb Cortex 1991; 1: 103–16.

3. Lee VMY, Balin BJ, Otvos LJ et al. A68: a major subunit of paired helical filaments and derivatized forms of normal tau. Science 1991; 251: 675–8.

4. Braak H, Braak E. Neuropathological staging of Alzheimer-related changes. Acta Neuropathol 1991; 82: 239–59.

5. Braak H, Braak E. Evolution of the neuropathology of Alzheimer's disease. Acta Neurol Scand 1996; 65(Suppl): 3–12.

6. Akiyama H, Barger S, Barnum S et al. Inflammation and Alzheimer's disease. Neurobiol Aging 2000; 21: 383–421.

7. Khachaturian ZS. Diagnosis of Alzheimer's disease. Arch Neurol 1985; 42: 1097–105.

8. Mirra SS, Heyman A, McKeel D et al. The consortium to establish a registry for Alzheimer's disease (CERAD). Part II. Standardization of the neuropathologic assessment of Alzheimer's disease. Neurology 1991; 41: 479–86.

9. The National Institute on Aging and Reagan Institute Working Group on Diagnostic Criteria for the Neuropathological Assessment of Alzheimer's Disease. Consensus recommendations for the postmortem diagnosis of Alzheimer's disease. Neurobiol Aging 1997; 18: S1–2.

10. Gearing M, Mirra SS, Hedreen JC et al. The consortium to establish a registry for Alzheimer's disease. Part X. Neuropathology confirmation of the clinical diagnosis of Alzheimer's disease. Neurology 1995; 45: 461–6.

11. Snowdon DA, Greiner LH, Mortimer JA et al. Brain infarction and the clinical expression of Alzheimer disease: the nun study. JAMA 1997; 277: 813–17.

12. Hardy J. Molecular genetics of Alzheimer's disease. Acta Neurol Scand 1996; 165: 13–17.

CHAPTER 6

Prevention of Alzheimer's disease

Claudia Jacova, Benita Mudge, and Michael Woodward

WHAT IS PREVENTION OF ALZHEIMER'S DISEASE

Preventive thinking in medicine has an ancient heritage but prevention science, with its empirical research and empirically grounded theories, has developed only in the latter part of the 20th century.[1] The application of preventive thinking to Alzheimer's disease (AD) is recent, with research still in its infancy at the beginning of the 21st century. The preventability of AD is stirring broad interest among researchers in the field because of the recognition that current approved treatments for AD have symptomatic but not disease-modifying effects (Figure 6.1).

AD is a chronic disease that typically begins in late life. It has been suggested that approaches to prevent AD will likely parallel those that are being developed for other chronic diseases of later life.[2] This chapter presents a summary of our knowledge about the prevention of AD, the lessons we have already learned, the hypotheses that are being pursued, and the challenges that future research will need to address before AD prevention programs can be considered for general application within the population.

Prevention comprises a spectrum of interventions. Figure 6.2 shows the application of the prevention spectrum to AD. *Primary* preventive measures are applied to the induction stage where early pathogenic processes begin to develop in the brains of those individuals that will eventually have AD. *Secondary* prevention occurs in the latency stage, clinically defined by questionable or mild symptoms known as mild cognitive impairment

(MCI),[4] with the accompanying pathologic processes now detectable on neuroimaging and neuropathology. The percentage of MCI cases that advance to AD is 10 to 15% per annum, compared to 1 to 2% for normal subjects.[5] The MCI stage is the ideal window for treatment of the earliest disease symptoms, with the aim of slowing the progression to full-blown disease. *Tertiary* prevention or treatment proper begins when MCI advances to AD, with its pathologic cascade of increasing amyloidopathy, tangle formation, neuronal death, and inflammatory changes.

Primary prevention of AD is currently focused on delaying the development of clinical symptoms and their progression to overt dementia rather than on intercepting the initial pathogenic event. The onset of neuropathologic changes in persons who later develop AD may occur decades before the disease becomes expressed.[6] Primary preventive interventions are therefore likely to be administered with prodromal pathology already in progress. But delaying the progression of the prodromal pathology and the onset of clinical symptoms would still be highly beneficial because it would enable many at-risk individuals to continue to function adequately into late life. In fact, individuals may die of other, non-AD causes before the devastating symptoms of dementia reach expression. Table 6.1 shows the estimated effect that interventions to delay the onset of AD would have on the number of people affected in the United States 10, 30, and 50 years later. If the onset of AD could be delayed by 5 years, the number of cases could be reduced by as much as 50% in 30 years.[7]

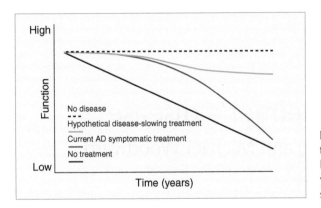

Figure 6.1 Different treatment effects in AD compared to no treatment and no disease. Current treatment approaches to AD have symptomatic but not disease-modifying effects. It may be years until treatments become available that are capable of slowing, halting, or even reversing AD.

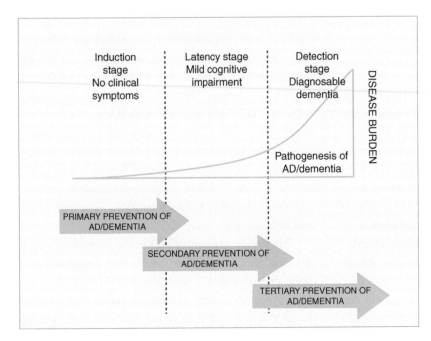

Figure 6.2 The spectrum of preventive approaches applied to the clinical stages of AD and to its pathogenesis. Boundaries between clinical stages are set somewhat arbitrarily and generate overlap between primary, secondary, and tertiary prevention. Adapted from[3] Figure 1. Reproduced with the permission of the publisher.

Table 6.1 The effects that interventions to delay the onset of AD might have on the prevalence of AD in the US population. Interventions are assumed to begin in 1998

Reduction in age-specific incidence (%)	Mean delay (years)	AD prevalence in 2007 (millions)	AD prevalence in 2027 (millions)	AD prevalence in 2047 (millions)
0	0	2.89	4.74	8.64
5	0.5	2.79	4.52	8.26
10	1.0	2.68	4.31	7.87
25	2.0	2.32	3.64	6.70
50	5.0	1.74	2.49	4.60

From [6] Table 2. Reprinted with permission from the American Public Health Association.

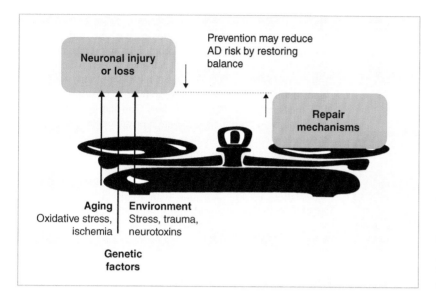

Figure 6.3 Brain aging and AD can be understood as an imbalance between neuronal injury triggered by normal age-related processes, genetic factors, and environmental exposures, and repair mechanisms. Preventive interventions may be able to correct this imbalance by reducing neuronal injury and by promoting repair mechanisms. Adapted from[8] Figure 1, © 2002, with permission from Elsevier.

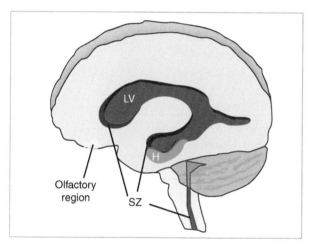

Figure 6.4 Neural stem cells in the adult human brain are found in the subependymal zone (red) lining the lateral ventricle, the subventricular zone (SZ) of the spinal cord (red), and the hippocampus (H) (green). Rodent brainstem cells migrate towards the olfactory region (yellow). This migratory pattern has not been firmly established within the adult human brain. Reprinted from [9] Figure 1, © 2004, with permission from Elsevier.

THE BIOLOGICAL PLAUSIBILITY OF AD PREVENTION

A question fundamental to all prevention research concerns which potential biological targets should be intervened on. Age- and AD-related changes in the brain can be envisioned as an imbalance between the increasing burden of neuronal injury consequent to normal aging processes, disease, trauma, and genetic factors, and a diminishing capacity of the mechanisms of repair.[8] Figure 6.3 illustrates the mechanisms involved in this imbalance, together with the two major pathways by which preventive interventions may correct the imbalance.

Modifying the factors that cause neuronal injury is one major pathway for AD prevention. While it may not yet be possible to manipulate genetic vulnerability, processes of biological aging, such as oxidative stress or cerebral vascular insufficiency, as well as environmental factors causing injury, are amenable to intervention. The other major pathway is the promotion of repair and regeneration mechanisms. A growing body of evidence in neuroscience research indicates that brain plasticity is retained to some extent throughout adult life. Animal studies have shown that the adult brain is capable of generating new neurons (see Figure 6.4), forging new connections among neurons, and enhancing its vasculature by adding new capillaries.[10] The potential for neurogenesis in the human brain is less well understood, in particular with regard to its impact on functional capacity.

Plasticity and repair mechanisms may support the lifelong accumulation of cognitive reserve, a set of skills and repertoires attributed to innate characteristics as well as to learning, experience, and activity patterns. High levels of cognitive reserve are believed to increase an individual's tolerance to AD pathology and prolong everyday functioning, even when there is advanced neurodegeneration.[11] Figure 6.5 shows evidence from a positron emission tomography (PET) study in support of the cognitive reserve hypothesis.

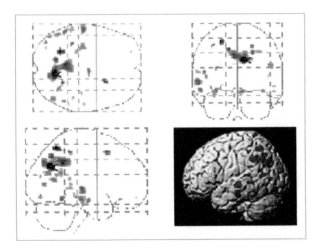

Figure 6.5 In a positron emission tomography (PET) study of patients with mild AD, cognitive reserve was estimated by measures of education, premorbid IQ, and engagement in intellectual, social, and physical activities. When patients were matched on the severity of their clinical symptoms, a negative association emerged between cognitive reserve measures and PET measures of cerebral blood flow. The statistical parametric brain maps and the 3-dimensional representation below depict the areas where these inverse associations were strongest. This study suggests people with high levels of cognitive reserve may better tolerate blood flow reductions and maintain functioning in the face of advancing AD pathology. From Scarmeas N et al. Association of life activities with cerebral blood flow in Alzheimer disease. Reproduced from[12] with the permission of the publisher.

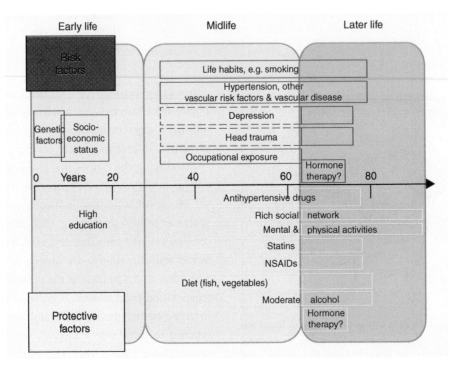

Figure 6.6 Risk and protective factors for AD may exert their most critical influence at different times in the life course of an individual. The timeline has been developed based on the age(s) for which associations have been reported in the epidemiologic literature. Dashed lines indicate hypothetical times of activity. The timeline highlights three key periods for risk/protective factors. Early life is likely most critical for the development of reserve (learning and education) but it may also be a time when distal adverse influences contributing to the risk of adult disease and later life AD first become active. Life habits, and the development and control of vascular and metabolic risk factors, become decisive in midlife (40s to 60s), whereas mental and physical activity patterns may continue to moderate the risk of AD into later life. Adapted from Fratiglioni et al. An active and socially integrated lifestyle in late life might protect against dementia. Lancet Neurology 2004; 3: 343–53,13 Figure 2, © 2004, with permission from Elsevier.

THE TIMING OF AD PREVENTION

When should prevention begin? At what life stage(s) are preventive interventions most effective? Is it ever too late to institute preventive measures? The best available answers to these questions currently stem from epidemiologic studies that have found associations between modifiable risk and protective factors, and the incidence of AD. These factors are known to have their most critical influence at different times in the life course of an individual. Figure 6.6 shows a timeline of risk and protective factors which has been developed based on the age(s) for which associations have been reported in the literature.[13]

Studies have shown that hypertension acts as an important risk factor in midlife but not near the time of

AD diagnosis. Treating hypertension during midlife may be more effective for AD prevention than treatment in later life. Similarly, estrogen plus progestin were unsuccessful in reducing the incidence of AD and other dementias in women aged 65 or older,[14] but it has been suggested that if treatment were initiated around menopause (10 years earlier), a positive treatment effect might be achieved.[15] By contrast, it is possible that interventions targeting lifestyle factors (cognitive, exercise, social network) may maintain robust effects through later life.

ASSESSING THE EVIDENCE ON AD PREVENTION

Self-help books, popular magazines, and web sites devoted to the maintenance of brain health may create the impression that strategies with established efficacy are already in hand. In reality our knowledge of what might work in AD prevention is preliminary, with the existing evidence derived primarily from observational studies that have investigated the relationship between exposure to putative risk factors and the probability of AD.

Observational studies have uncovered a rich network of life circumstances that are associated with the risk of developing AD. These circumstances range from psychosocial characteristics, to health and medical conditions, to exposure to certain environmental events, and use of pharmacologic agents. Observational studies have succeeded in pinpointing positive risk factors, that is factors associated with an increased occurrence of AD in those exposed to them, and negative risk factors or protective factors, where exposure is associated with a reduced rate of AD. Tables 6.2 and 6.3 list modifiable

Table 6.2 Modifiable protective factors for AD

Possible	Unlikely
Leisure/social activities	Symptomatic drugs for AD (cholinesterase inhibitors)
Physical activity	Vitamin E intake
Ongoing intellectual stimulation	
Higher education	
Moderate alcohol intake	
Anti-inflammatory drugs	
Omega-3-fatty acid intake	
Ginkgo biloba	

Table 6.3 Modifiable risk factors for AD

Likely	Uncertain	Unlikely
Vascular risk factors including	Elevated homocysteine/low	Hormone replacement therapy/
• Smoking	B12 and folate	estrogen
• Diabetes	Cholesterol-lowering drugs	Strong exposure to electromagnetic
• Obesity	Depression	radiation
• Hypertension	Sleep disorders	Aluminum and other metallic ions
• Cardiac bypass surgery		
• Metabolic syndrome		
Head injury		

protective and risk factors for AD according to the strength of the currently available evidence.

Risk factor information provides a wealth of leads on interventions that might work to prevent AD but, where possible, rigorous testing of these interventions through randomized controlled trials (RCTs) is needed before they can be scientifically accepted. All observational studies have common fundamental limitations that preclude direct application of their findings to preventive programs. An association between two phenomena, for example use of antioxidant vitamin supplements and reduced risk of AD, cannot be taken as evidence of a causal link even if vitamin use is shown to have occurred before the onset of AD. The interpretive dilemma presenting itself to researchers who deal with evidence based on an association is illustrated in Figure 6.7.

RCTs provide the definitive test for the preventive effect of a treatment, but they pose significant feasibility, cost, and treatment safety issues when primary prevention is the objective, with its natural focus on essentially healthy study populations. Trials of this type require very large sample sizes and long observation periods to accrue sufficient numbers of incident AD cases for comparison of treatment and placebo arms. At the time

of writing, eight primary prevention of AD or dementia trials have been designed and implemented in the US and Europe (Table 6.4). The size and cost of these trials have not been their only difficulty. Three trials had to be discontinued because the treatments - with estrogen and progestin and with non-steroidal anti-inflammatory drugs (NSAIDs) - involved health risks unacceptable in primary prevention. It is clear that, while many more trials are needed to create a sufficient knowledge base for preventive programs, a key concern will be the risk of any intervention, which must be minimal when targeting healthy individuals.

The first primary prevention RCTs have been designed to test non-steroidal anti-inflammatory drugs, hormonal therapy, antihypertensive drugs, antioxidants, and supplements. Many other epidemiologic leads exist but not all are worth pursuing as candidate interventions in AD prevention. First, candidate interventions should have biological plausibility. Second, the interventions must involve minimal risk for healthy normal individuals and an acceptable risk-benefit ratio when given to individuals at identified risk of AD. Third, the intervention should be affordable and acceptable to people. Sustained changes in behavior are possible if there is

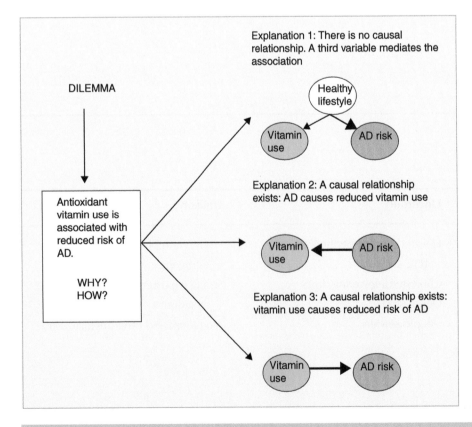

Figure 6.7 When associations between the exposure to a risk/protective factor and AD incidence are found, no causal inferences can be made. By design, observational studies cannot control for a host of circumstances, characteristics, or conditions that might be responsible for the association. Even if it were possible to rule out the influence of all confounding factors, the direction of the relationship between the risk factor and AD would remain elusive.

Table 6.4 The first generation of primary prevention RCTs comprises eight trials. Three trials have been discontinued because the treatments were not deemed sufficiently safe

Trial (Acronym)	Status	Intervention	Subject selection criteria	Duration (years)	Overall estimated incidence rate (% per year)	Planned sample size
PREPARE	Discontinued	Conjugated equine estrogen alone; Conj equ estrogen + medroxyprogesterone acetate	Female sex, Family history of AD, Age ≥ 65	3	5	900
ADAPT	Discontinued	Naproxen or celecoxib	Family history of dementia, Age ≥ 70	5–7	3–3.4	2 800
SYST-EUR	Completed	Nitrendipine and/or enalapril and/or hydrochlorothiazide	Systolic hypertension, Age ≥ 60	5	1.6	3 000
SCOPE	Completed	Candesartan cilexetil	Systolic hypertension, Age 70 to 89	3–5	2.4	4 000
GEMS	Ongoing extended	*Ginkgo biloba*	Age ≥ 75 (≥ 71 if of African ancestry)	5	4	3 000
GUIDAGE	Ongoing	*Ginkgo biloba*	Age ≥ 70, Memory complaints	5	2.4	2 800
WHIMS	Discontinued	Conjugated equine estrogen alone; Conj equ estrogen + medroxypro-gesterone acetate	Female sex, Age ≥ 65	6	2	8 300
PREADVISE	Ongoing	Vitamin E or selenium or both	Age ≥ 62 (≥ 60 if of African or Hispanic ancestry)	9–12	1	10 700

Reprinted from [16] with the permission of the publisher.

sufficient awareness of the importance of the intervention, but long-term compliance with a medication, possibly with side-effects, is unlikely.

CANDIDATE INTERVENTIONS FOR AD PREVENTION

Interventions targeting vascular risk factors

AD and vascular types of dementia share many risk factors. For example, genetic predisposition including the apolipoprotein E genotype is implicated both in AD and vascular disease. Vascular pathology is often found in AD, as shown in Figure 6.8. Interventions on vascular risk factors hold substantial promise in AD prevention as they may have the added advantage of protecting from vascular types of dementia as well as from cardiovascular disease.

Hypertension and stroke

The most extensively studied risk factor in the context of AD prevention has been hypertension. Several RCTs, with mean follow-up times approaching 4 years, provide evidence that antihypertensive medications can reduce the incidence of AD and cognitive impairment in subjects who are at increased risk because of hypertension or cerebrovascular disease. Figure 6.9 shows the key findings from three of these RCTs. In the Syst-Eur study (panel a) the calcium-channel blocker nitrendipine reduced incident cases of AD and other dementias by 55%.[18] In the HOPE study (panel b) the angiotensin-converting enzyme (ACE) inhibitor ramipril reduced the risk of cognitive impairment.[19] The PROGRESS study (panel c) found that perindropril (also an ACE inhibitor) provided protection against cognitive decline and dementia in people who suffered a stroke during the follow-up period of the trial.[20] Additionally, the Study on Cognition and Prognosis in the Elderly (SCOPE) has shown that candesartan (an angiotensin blocker) slowed decline in non-demented subjects whose cognitive performance at study entry was mildly impaired.[21] Syst-Eur and SCOPE targeted age groups 65 years or older, thus suggesting that the treatment of hypertension may be an effective preventive strategy, even when administered in later rather than midlife.

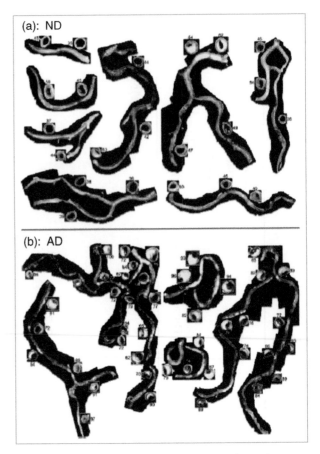

(a): ND

(b): AD

Figure 6.8 There is known overlap between cerebrovascular disease and AD. A neuropathologic study compared atherosclerosis of the leptomeningeal arteries in autopsy cases of AD and normal elderly. Mean degree of occlusion was greater in arteries of AD cases. The diagram shows arterial cross-sections from a normal control (ND) and an AD case. Arterial occlusions were extensive and severe in the AD case, with those boxed in red .90%. Figure 1, p. 2625. Reproduced from[17] with the permission of the publisher.

Stroke is a known risk factor for AD. Several studies have shown that atherosclerosis and other stroke risk factors are also risk factors for AD. In the Nun study, a longitudinal study of aging and AD that included Catholic convent sisters aged 75 to 106 years, the presence of brain infarcts was associated with a higher incidence of AD and with more severe clinical symptoms.[22] The HOPE and PROGRESS studies both found that antihypertensive medications lower the incidence of cognitive decline in those at high risk of or having had a stroke, even in the absence of hypertension. These studies support both the treatment of hypertension as well as the lowering of blood pressure in those at increased risk of stroke.

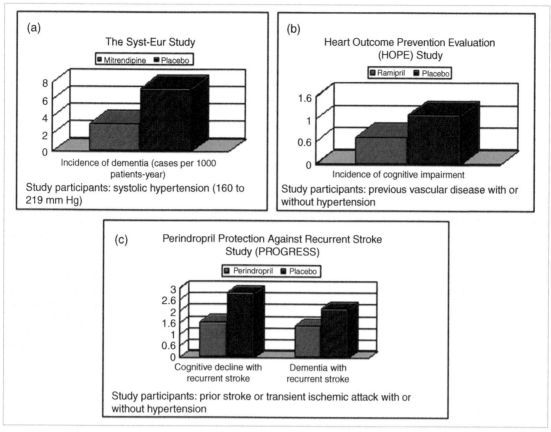

Figure 6.9 The effects of treatment with antihypertensive medication on risk of dementia and cognitive impairment have been studied in 3 RCTs: The Systolic Hypertension in Europe (Syst-Eur) Study, 2002,[18] the Heart Outcome Prevention Evaluations (Hope) Study, 2002,[19] and the Perindropril Protection Against Recurrent Stroke (PROGRESS) Study, 1996.[20] The panels in the figure each present the consistently positive results that these trials have achieved. All trials have involved subjects with hypertension and/or increased risk of stroke.

Other approaches to reduce the risk of stroke may also reduce the risk of AD, but this has yet to be demonstrated.

Diabetes mellitus

Numerous studies have shown a link between hyperinsulinemia, and cognitive decline and AD. It might be anticipated that tight control of blood sugar in diabetes mellitus would reduce the incidence and possibly the rate of decline of AD; however, there is no evidence yet to support this idea. Trials with antidiabetic drugs known as the glitazones (thiazolidenediones) are under way, but these drugs may have effects on AD pathogenesis that are independent of control of blood glucose.[23] The potential of antidiabetic medication as a candidate treatment in AD prevention remains to be investigated.

Cholesterol

A number of retrospective case-control studies reported that the use of cholesterol-lowering agents known as statins (hydroxy-methylglutaryl-coenzyme A reductase inhibitors) was associated with a risk reduction of AD ranging from 44 to 71%. More recent prospective cohort studies, however, have not found similar associations. Two large recent statin RCTs with normal subjects have failed to demonstrate any cognitive treatment benefit or reduction in the incidence of AD (a secondary outcome).[24,25] The potential of statins as primary prevention agents remains to be fully assessed. Because cholesterol has been hypothesized to modulate the processing of amyloid precursor protein and the transportation of the amyloid beta peptide,[26] there is a rationale for pursuing statins in the context of AD prevention.

Dietary fat intake

The intake of unsaturated, unhydrogenated fats has been found to reduce the risk for AD, while the intake of saturated or trans-unsaturated fats has been associated with an increased risk.[27] Animal models of AD have suggested that a diet enriched with omega-3 polyunsaturated fatty acids reduces amyloid burden.[28] These fatty acids are found in some types of fish and seafood and, in fact, large prospective cohort studies have shown an association between fish intake and risk for dementia. For example, a study in south-western France that followed normal elderly over 7 years, showed that those eating fish or seafood at least once a week had a >30% reduced risk of dementia.[29] Dietary or supplement intake of 'good' fats has yet to be tested in a prevention RCT, but it is recommended because of its broader health benefits.

Caloric intake and body weight

Midlife obesity appears to increase the risk of later dementia. In a study of men and women initially aged 40–45 and followed from a baseline evaluation in 1964–73 to 1994, initially obese individuals had a 74% increased risk of dementia.[30] There have been similar findings for later life obesity. These observations are consistent with dietary interventions in animal models of AD, where caloric restriction and intermittent fasting have been found to protect neurons against AD degenerative processes.[31] There may also be danger in excessive weight loss, with several studies linking undernutrition and declining body mass to AD.[32] In these studies, however, it is not clear whether weight loss is a very early symptom of dementia rather than having a causal role. Because avoidance of over- and undernutrition has broader health benefits, it is advisable even though direct effects on dementia risk remain uncertain.

Pharmacologic interventions

Estrogen

At least 16 observational studies have shown an association for estrogen therapy and a reduced risk of AD. In one study of elderly women initially free of AD, estrogen therapy was associated with a 60% reduction in the development of AD 5 years later.[33] It has also been suggested that estrogen may improve memory in cognitively normal women, but a systematic review of trials has concluded that there is little evidence of beneficial effects.[34] In the Women's Health Initiative Study (WHIMS), women aged 65 to 79 years, initially free of dementia, failed to benefit from treatment with estrogen and progestin or with estrogen alone, and were 40 to 100% more likely than women receiving placebo to develop cognitive impairment and dementia.[14,35] Both treatments in this trial have been halted because of increased health risks. The WHIMS experience underscores the potential dangers in adapting interventions from observational studies without subjecting them to rigorous tests.

The Multiple Outcomes of Raloxifene Evaluation (MORE) study of postmenopausal women with osteoporosis has produced only slightly more encouraging results. Raloxifene, a selective estrogen receptor modulator, reduced the risk of developing mild cognitive impairment by >30% but had no significant benefit on the development of AD and other dementias.[36] At this time, hormone replacement therapy cannot be recommended for the prevention of AD, though research may still be warranted to investigate interventions earlier in the lifecycle.

Anti-inflammatory agents

Epidemiologic studies have consistently shown a relationship between the use of non-steroidal anti-inflammatory drugs (NSAIDs) and reduced risk of dementia. The size of risk reduction is related to the duration of cumulative NSAID use, as shown in Figure 6.10. A systematic review and meta-analysis of observational

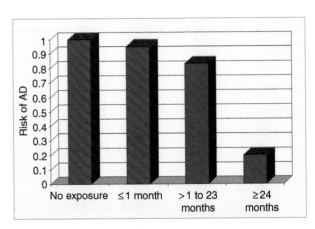

Figure 6.10 In the Rotterdam study, a large prospective cohort study of people 55 years of age or older, risk reduction for AD due to NSAIDs was dependent on the cumulative duration of use. While short-term use (≤1 month) was not beneficial, use for 2 years or longer reduced risk by 80%. These data have been reported by In't Veld et al.[38]

studies showed a pooled risk reduction of roughly 30% among NSAID users.[37]

The observational evidence fits with established knowledge that there is inflammation in the brains of those with AD, including accumulation of microglia around plaques, a local cytokine-mediated acute-phase response, and the activation of the complement cascade.[38] On this basis the hypothesis has been advanced that NSAIDs may be useful in reducing the risk of AD and in treating established AD. Unfortunately, large trials published to date have failed to show a consistent beneficial effect of NSAID therapy in established AD.[39] Failure to benefit established AD does not, however, mean there will be an equal lack of success in preventing the disease. The AD Anti-Inflammatory Prevention Trial (ADAPT) commenced in 2001 to test the efficacy of naproxen and celecoxib. This trial was suspended in 2004, after participants had been treated for only up to 3 years, due to increased cardiovascular and stroke risk in those receiving naproxen. At the same time other large trials were raising concerns about the safety of celecoxib.[40] ADAPT participants will be followed up to see if even the relatively short exposure reduces the incidence of AD, and to further evaluate the long-term safety of this exposure. At this time, anti-inflammatory drugs cannot be recommended as primary prevention agents and increasing safety concerns make their use in a healthy population unlikely. The ADAPT experience raises important questions about what constitutes an acceptable risk-benefit ratio in the treatment of normal individuals, and how this ratio may change as an individual's risk of AD increases.

Cholinesterase inhibitors

Acetylcholinesterase inhibitors (AChEIs) represent the main therapeutic approach to the symptoms of AD. Several trials have tested their efficacy in people with mild cognitive impairment (MCI), a condition intermediate between normal aging and AD. Results in the long term have generally been disappointing, where treatment with donepezil, rivastigmine, or galantamine did not significantly slow rates of progression to AD in MCI patients.[41–43] It was noteworthy that carriers of the apolipoprotein "4 allele treated with donepezil appeared to derive sustained benefits, as shown in Figure 6.11.[41] It is generally regarded as appropriate to discuss AChEIs with patients with MCI, but at this stage, clinicians are not recommending that these drugs be used to treat MCI, and in no country have regulatory authorities approved its use in MCI.

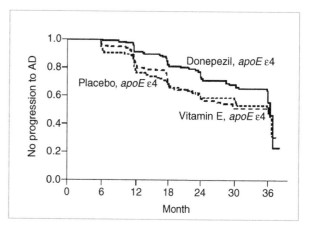

Figure 6.11 In a large RCT of donepezil in mild cognitive impairment, a condition at high risk of progression to AD, there were no overall differences in 3-year progression rates between those receiving treatment and those receiving placebo. There was, however, a sustained benefit among carriers of one or two apoE ε4 alleles: donepezil reduced their risk of progression to AD by approximately one-third at year 3. From [41]Figure 1(D). Reproduced with the permission of the Massachusetts Medical Society.

Vitamins and complementary medications

Vitamin B12, folate, and homocysteine

Numerous studies have shown an association between dementia risk, low intake of vitamin B12 and folate, and elevated levels of homocysteine. These factors are associated with cognitive decline also in the absence of dementia. One of the first prospective studies to draw attention to B12 and folate was the Kungsholmen Project, where subjects with low levels had twice the risk of developing dementia compared to subjects with normal levels of these vitamins.[44] Homocysteine levels may be a risk factor for dementia as they are for cardiovascular disease. Indeed, increased cardiovascular risk may be the link between elevated homocysteine and dementia. Higher homocysteine has been associated with the presence of brain white matter changes (leukoariosis) in AD,[45] and with cerebral small vessel disease in non-demented people.[46]

As seen in Figure 6.12, homocysteine is an intermediate product in the methionine cycle whose metabolism is dependent on B12 and folate. Hence, maintenance of adequate B12 and folate intake, or routine supplementation, could prevent cognitive decline and dementia. A recent unpublished study reported that 0.8 mg daily of folate protected against cognitive decline in subjects who

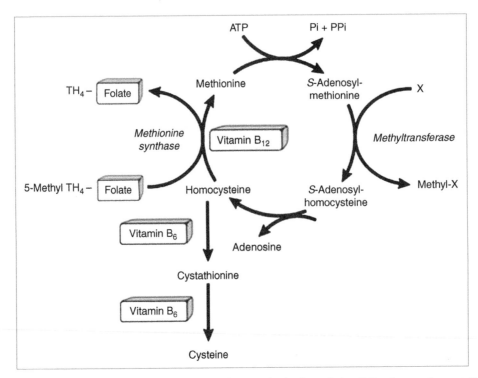

Figure 6.12 The methionine–homocysteine–folate–B12 cycle provides biological plausibility for supplementation with vitamin B12 and folate. Homocysteine is an intermediate product in the metabolism of the amino acid methionine. Homocysteine is remethylated to methionine by a folate-dependent reaction, which in turn is catalyzed by methionine synthase, a vitamin B12 dependent enzyme. Insufficient availability of B12 and/or folate may lead to build-up of homocysteine. From Biological methylation reactions and homocysteine metabolism, accessed from the Linus Pauling Institute website http://lpi.oregonstate.edu/infocenter/vitamins/vitaminB12/figure9_1.html on 19 April 2006. Reprinted with permission from the Linus Pauling Institute.

did not have folate deficiency.[47] These results need to be replicated but, as supplementation with folate is generally safe, it is likely that its supplementation will become a practice norm even before such data are available.

Vitamins E and C

AD is characterized by neuropathology that may in part be mediated by oxidative damage. It is therefore possible that vitamins with antioxidant effects, including E and C, have a protective effect.

The Rotterdam study assessed its participants' dietary intake of vitamins E and C and found an almost 20% lowered risk of AD for every 1 standard deviation increase in these vitamins. Risk reduction was statistically significant for vitamin C and borderline for vitamin E.[48] The Chicago Health and Aging Project found a strong risk reduction of AD due to increased dietary vitamin E intake, but only among persons who were apolipoprotein ε4 negative. Supplementation with vitamins C and E was not associated with a lower risk.[49] In the large donepezil trial in MCI, a vitamin E arm of treatment had no effect on the rate of progression to AD.[41]

Vitamin E does not appear to have preventive efficacy. Safety concerns have recently emerged, with vitamin E use being linked to higher rates of mortality.[50] On this basis, vitamin E cannot be recommended at any dose for AD prevention.

Ginkgo biloba

Ginkgo biloba extract is widely prescribed throughout the world to memory-impaired people. Its effects are antioxidant and blood flow enhancing. Given its popularity and near universal acceptance, attention has focused on its potential as a preventive agent. RCTs designed to directly assess its efficacy are in progress (GEMS, GuidAge). At this stage there is no evidence to recommend *Ginkgo biloba* as a preventive agent.

Lifestyle interventions

Leisure and social activities

There is enormous public interest in the role that lifestyle factors play in maintaining cognitive function and protecting against dementia. Epidemiologic studies have fuelled this interest further by reporting associations between the range and intensity of leisure and social activities, and the risk of dementia, Because very early AD may have an impact on activity patterns and interests, it is especially important in this context to be mindful of the limitations of the evidence. Cognitive engagement may stimulate synaptogenic processes that protect against dementia, but it is also possible that people are more engaged cognitively because they do not have preclinical AD. Statistical adjustment for baseline cognitive functioning, or analysis limited to subjects who remained dementia free for a substantial time after enrolment, have been strategies to address this problem, but they still do not allow for causal inferences to be drawn.

Table 6.5 shows a summary of activity measurement methods and findings from two large prospective cohort

Table 6.5 Two large prospective cohort studies have found an association between high levels of leisure/cognitive activities and reduced AD risk

The Washington Heights–Inwood aging project[51]	The Bronx aging study[52]

THE ACTIVITY SCORE:
Self-reported participation in activities over the previous month:
 	
    Knitting, music or other hobby
    Walking for pleasure or excursion*
    Visiting friends or relatives*
    Being visited by friends or relatives
    Physical conditioning
    Going to movies, restaurants, or sporting events*
    Reading newspapers, magazines, or books*
    Watching television or listening to the radio
    Doing community volunteer work
    Playing cards, games, or bingo
    Going to a club or center
    Going to classes
    Going to church, synagogue, or temple
Score = Total points received, with 1 point/activity.
	THE ACTIVITY SCORES:
	Frequency of participation in activities (daily = 7; several days per week = 4; once weekly = 1; monthly, occasionally, never = 0):
	Cognitive activities:
	    Reading books or newspapers*
	    Writing for pleasure
	    Doing crossword puzzles
	    Playing board games or cards*
	    Participating in organized group discussions
	    Playing a musical instrument*
	Score = Total points received, with 1 point = 1 activity/day/week
	
	Physical activities:
	    Dancing*
	    Doing housework
	    Walking for exercise
	    Climbing stairs
	    Bicycling
	    Swimming
	    Playing team games
	    Playing tennis or golf
	    Group exercises
	    Babysitting
	Score = Total points received, with 1 point = 1 activity/day/week

The Finding:
A high activity score is associated with a reduced risk of AD:
 	
    Scores > 6 are associated with 38% risk reduction
	The Findings:
	High cognitive but not physical activity scores are associated with reduced risk of AD:
	
	Compared to a cognitive activity score < 8:
	    Scores 8–11 risk reduction 50%
	    Scores > 11 risk reduction 67%

*Activities most strongly associated with reduced risk	*Activities most strongly associated with reduced risk

studies that have followed subjects initially free of dementia for a number of years. Both studies suggest that people with high levels of activity have a reduced risk of AD.[51,52] Estimates of risk reduction have ranged from 38 to 67%. In one study a 'dose' effect of activity emerged, with higher activity levels associated with larger risk reductions than intermediate levels.[52] The associations remained even when baseline cognitive performance, health limitations interfering with desired leisure activities, cerebrovascular disease, and depression were considered, or when only subjects developing dementia after more than 7 years were included. Some activities may have a stronger protective effect than others (Figure 6.13), but because the two studies have utilized different measures, cross-comparisons and generalizations are not possible.

The promotion of a healthy and socially active lifestyle is highly unlikely to be associated with harm and can be encouraged. To establish a scientific basis, which could support public policy and expenditure, lifestyle interventions for the prevention of AD should be tested in RCTs. This type of RCT is possible in principle. Table 6.6 shows examples of 'placebo' conditions that have been utilized in trials of lifestyle interventions to improve cognition.

Physical activity

There is growing evidence from animal studies that exercise can enhance brain structure and function.[9] Human studies have documented a link between physical activity and cognitive function. In the Women Who Walk Study, baseline physical activity was measured as self-reported 160 m units of walking and then divided into quartiles. Women whose physical activity score fell in the highest quartile had a 34% reduced risk of cognitive decline compared to women in the lowest quartile.[56] In the Nurses' Health Study women completed questionnaires on their physical activities beginning in 1986 and received telephone cognitive assessments from 1995 to 2001. Women in the highest quintile of physical activity had a 20% lower risk of cognitive impairment than women in the lowest quintile. Those performing the equivalent of walking at an easy pace for at least 1.5 hours/week had higher cognitive scores than those walking less than 40 minutes/week.[57] There is also RCT evidence that physical activity programs can benefit

(a)

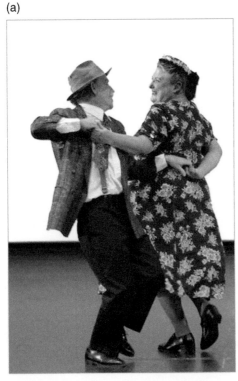

(b)

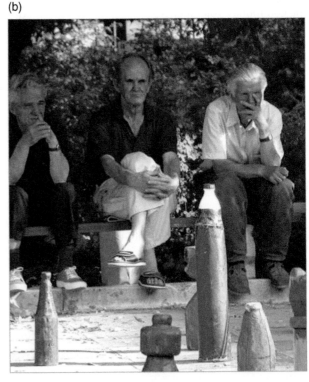

Figure 6.13 A research team from the Albert Einstein College of Medicine, Bronx, NY[52] found that participation in leisure activities is associated with a reduced risk of dementia. People who engaged at least several times per week in dancing and in playing board games had a risk of AD and other dementias that was over 70% lower than that among people who engaged rarely in these activities.

Table 6.6 Placebo conditions employed in three cognitive or physical activity RCTs targeting normal elderly or patients with mild AD

Study	Active treatment	Placebo condition
Kramer et al 1999[53]	Aerobic exercise (walking)	Anaerobic exercise (stretching and toning)
Cahn-Weiner et al 2003[54]	Six sessions consisting of memory training in word recall and recognition and mnemonic strategies to enhance memory and organizational skills	Six sessions consisting of presentations of educational information pertaining to aging and dementia but no formal memory training
Davis et al 2001[55]	Weekly visits consisting of training in spaced retrieval, word recall, face–name associations, and at-home cognitive stimulation exercises	Weekly visits consisting of unstructured conversation and questioning by examiner Participants recited over learned material (e.g. alphabet, months of the year and days of the week) and watched videotapes on general health issues

cognitive test performance in older persons.[58,59] The Canadian Study of Health and Aging found a 30% reduction in the risk of AD associated with regular physical activity,[60] but other large cohort studies did not find similar risk reductions.[52,61] On balance, there is support for a role for physical activity in AD prevention but no definitive proof. However, physical activity can be strongly recommended because, in addition to its putative direct effects on brain neurogenesis and angiogenesis, it may protect from AD indirectly by maintaining cardiovascular health.

Alcohol and smoking

Both alcohol and smoking have been proposed to protect from dementia, though each has both positive and negative potential. For example, nicotine can stimulate cholinergic neurotransmission, but it also accelerates atherosclerosis. Red wine may have some antioxidant properties, but it is also a depressant of the central nervous system.

Recent methodologically improved studies of smoking have demonstrated that it is not protective and that smokers are twice as likely to develop AD as non-smokers,[62] while recent studies of alcohol use have consistently supported the earlier identified protective effect of light-to-moderate consumption. In the Rotterdam study, intake of one to three alcoholic drinks per day was associated with a >40% lowered risk of any dementia.[63] In the US Cardiovascular Health Study, consumption of one to six drinks weekly was associated

with a >50% risk reduction.[64] This protective effect may be due to a reduction of cardiovascular risk factors via effects on platelets or lipid profile, or to increased release of acetylcholine. On balance, alcohol remains an intervention with both a clear up- and downside, for which only limited endorsement can be provided.

Other interventions to prevent AD

Aluminum exposure

Aluminum has been an AD risk factor of interest since the 1960s. Though it is clearly recognized to be neurotoxic, there has been no sustained and converging evidence that it is causative of AD or associated with significantly increased AD risk.[65] In a notorious industrial incident described in Figure 6.14, subjects exposed to aluminum sulfate did develop disturbances in cerebral function in the short term, but have not been found to have an increased risk of AD.

Electromagnetic radiation

Occupational exposure to electromagnetic radiation may place people at increased risk of AD. Occupations involving such exposure include seamstress, arc welding, and those using other unshielded electric motors. One case-control study found that the risk of AD was almost 4-fold in those exposed to strong electromagnetic radiation,[66] but others have failed to find similar evidence.[67] A reasonable but not essential precaution at this point would be to shield electrical

Water poisons thousands - 8 July, 1988

In the worst mass water poisoning in the UK, more than 20 tonnes of aluminum sulfate were accidentally tipped into the wrong reservoir at the Lowermoor Water Treatment Works in Camelford, North Cornwall. The driver was a contractor's relief driver who was unfamiliar with the unmanned plant layout and delivery procedure. The 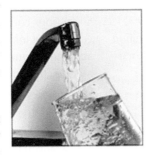 resulting acidic water directly entered the town's water supply and dissolved further contaminants from the antiquated distribution system including lead and copper. Despite numerous complaints from customers about the taste and cloudiness of the water, no warning was issued by the water authority until the following day. Subsequent complaints have included skin irritation and rashes, arthritic pain, sore throats, memory loss and general exhaustion and significant pressure from those affected for a public inquiry...

Figure 6.14 The Camelford water incident exposed thousands of people to aluminum sulfate in the drinking water. While neurotoxicity and brain dysfunction were observed in those exposed to the substance, there have been no reports of increased risk of AD. Water tap picture reproduced with the permission of the Water Efficiency Program, Toronto, ON, Canada.

motors whenever possible, especially when exposure is prolonged. Future research is likely to address whether the radiofrequency emissions from mobile phones (cellular and cordless) may contribute to AD risk.

Head injury

Head injury has often been evaluated as a risk factor of AD, with evidence that is quite mixed, as studies both support and refute a putative relationship between head injury and AD. In a study of World War II veterans who had a documented non-penetrating head injury during war service, the risk of AD was twice that of veterans who had not suffered head injuries. For severe head injury with loss of consciousness, the risk was 4-fold.[68] In the Rotterdam Study, however, no increased risk of AD was found for people who had a history of head trauma with loss of consciousness. No association emerged when multiple episodes of head trauma, time since head trauma, or duration of loss of consciousness were considered.[69] A meta-analysis of case-control studies indicated a small but significant effect of head injury on AD,[70] but a pooled sample analysis from four population-based studies in Europe did not.[71] Public interventions to forestall head trauma by imposing speed limits and the use of helmets and seatbelts are in place in many countries.

Education and occupation

Both educational and occupational achievement may enable individuals to accumulate cognitive reserve, thus offering protection from AD. In the Kungsholmen study, both high education and occupation levels reduced the risk of dementia when examined individually, but only education remained a significant factor when both were included in the analysis.[72] Most studies that have examined the association between education alone and dementia risk show a clear protective effect of higher educational achievement. In the Nurses' Health Study, women with an advanced degree (masters or doctoral) were >50% less likely, and women with a bachelor's degree 17% less likely to score poorly on a telephone-administered cognitive measure. Other socio-economic factors such as household income showed little or no association with cognitive function.[73] Regarding occupation, the evidence is less clear-cut. In a case-control study, the AD group's mental occupational demands were significantly lower than those of controls, whereas their physical occupational demands were comparable to controls.[74] In the PAQUID study, however, no association was found between occupation and the risk of AD.[75] While there is no practical or proven preventive strategy arising from these studies, it seems that mental activity may accumulate protective benefits in all stages of an individual's life course, in the form of higher education in young adulthood, as a mentally demanding occupation in mid-adulthood, and as leisure and social activities in later adulthood.

PUBLIC POLICY AND HEALTH PROMOTION

Public awareness and education will play a pivotal role in making the prevention of AD possible. Preventive strategies applicable to the general population will likely focus on lifestyle modification, including dietary,

(a)

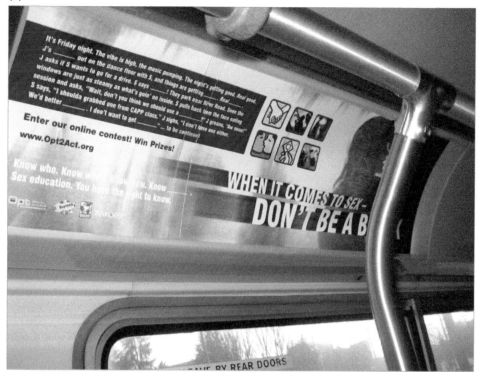

(b)

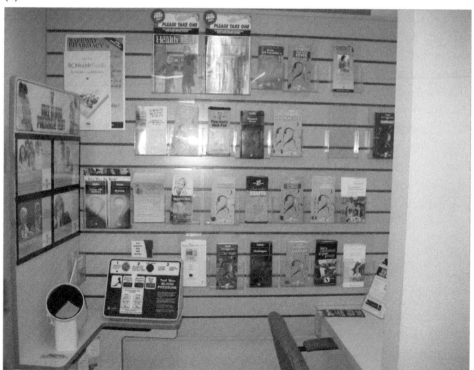

Figure 6.15 When population-wide interventions to prevent AD are proposed, the question of how to disseminate the relevant information and support people through lifestyle changes becomes important. Traditionally, health-promotional programs have been advertised on television, in pharmacies and doctors' offices, and on public transport. Computer technology may offer innovative approaches. The US Alzheimer's Association has launched a web-based information campaign (see Figure 6.16). In 2002, Health Canada began the E-Quit program to help people stop smoking with the support of daily e-mails (http://www.hc-sc.gc.ca/hl-vs/tobac-tabac/quit-cesser/now-maintenant/equit-jarrete/index_e.html, accessed on 30 January 2006). Perhaps this personalized approach may also find utility in AD prevention in the future.

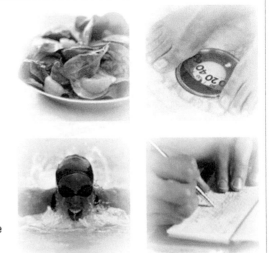

Think About Your Future.
Maintain Your Brain Today.

When people think about staying fit, they generally think from the neck down. But the health of your brain plays a critical role in almost everything you do: thinking, feeling, remembering, working, and playing – even sleeping.

The good news is that we now know there's a lot you can do to help keep your brain healthier as you age. These steps might also reduce your risk of Alzheimer's disease or other dementia.

Simple lifestyle modifications also would have an enormous impact on our nation's public health and the cost of healthcare. If you make brain-healthy lifestyle changes and take action by getting involved, we could realize a future without Alzheimer's disease.

The Alzheimer's Association Maintain Your Brain® materials and sub-brand logo are protected by trademark and copyright. The Maintain Your Brain® information and graphics used on this web site are not available for reprinting or repurposing by any organization other than the Alzheimer's Association and its chapter offices.

Figure 6.16 The US Alzheimer's Association has developed a preventive campaign that is posted on the web and is being disseminated through community workshops. From http://www.alz.org/maintainyourbrain/overview.asp, accessed 9 January, 2006. Reproduced with the permission of the Alzheimer's Association.

physical, and cognitive activity patterns, and possibly the use of non-prescription remedies. The success of these strategies will rely on the willingness of individuals to initiate and maintain behavioral change to delay the possible onset of AD in later life. It will be important to investigate effective ways to promote widespread awareness of AD risk and protective factors, and to support people through appropriate community health programs, products, and services (Figure 6.15). An early example of this type of initiative is the Maintain Your Brain® How to Live a Brain Healthy Lifestyle campaign initiated by the US Alzheimer's Association[76] (Figure 6.16).

CONCLUSION

The idea that AD can be prevented might have seemed a distant, almost unthinkable, outcome a mere decade ago. Now, at the beginning of the 21st century, delaying the devastating symptoms of AD is becoming a realistic goal thanks to relentless progress in the identification of AD risk factors and their treatment. Preventive strategies directed at controling vascular risk have already been proven effective, whereas other strategies including pharmacologic approaches, vitamin and dietary interventions, and lifestyle changes are being developed.

Risk factor modification has had a huge impact on cardiovascular health: total cardiovascular disease, heart disease, and stroke all declined in the latter part of the 20th century.[77] These improvements in cardiovascular health, along with other preventive strategies, are likely to reduce AD prevalence and incidence in the first decades of the 21st century. It may well turn out that future epidemiologic studies will report a time-lagged parallelism between declining cardiovascular disease and AD.

REFERENCES

1. Gullotta TP, Bloom M. Encyclopedia of Primary Prevention and Health Promotion. New York: Kluwer Academic/ Plenum Publishers 2003.

2. Larson EB, Kukull WA. Prevention of Alzheimer disease: a perspective based on successes in the prevention of other chronic diseases. Alzheimer Dis Assoc Disord 1996; 10(Suppl): 9–12.

3. Sano M. Noncholinergic treatment options for Alzheimer's disease. J Clin Psychiatry 2003; 64(Suppl 9): 23–8.

4. Petersen RC, Smith GE, Waring SC et al. Mild cognitive impairment: clinical characterization and outcome. Arch Neurol 1999; 56: 303-8.

5. Feldman HH, Jacova C. Mild cognitive impairment. Am J Geriatr Psychiatry 2005; 13(8): 645–55.

6. Braak H, Braak E. Neuropathological staging of Alzheimer-related changes. Acta Neuropathol (Berl) 1991; 82: 239–59.

7. Brookmeyer R, Gray S, Kawas C. Projections of Alzheimer's disease in the United States and the public health impact of delaying disease onset. Am J Public Health 1998; 88: 1337–42.

8. Ball LJ, Birge SJ. Prevention of brain aging and dementia. Clin Geriatr Med 18(3): 485–503.

9. Brazel C, Rao MS. Aging and neuronal replacement. Ageing Research Reviews 2004; 3: 465–83.

10. Churchill JD, Galvez R, Colcombe S et al. Exercise, experience and the aging brain. Neurobiol Aging 2002; 23(5): 941–55.

11. Stern Y. What is cognitive reserve? Theory and research application of the reserve concept. J Int Neuropsychol Soc 2002; 8(3): 448–60.

12. Scarmeas N, Zarahn E, Anderson KE et al. Association of life activities with cerebral blood flow in Alzheimer disease. Arch Neurol 2003; 60: 359–65.

13. Fratiglioni L, Paillard–Borg S, Winblad B. An active and socially integrated lifestyle in late life might protect against dementia. Lancet Neurol 2004; 3: 343–53.

14. Shumaker SA, Legault C, Thal L et al. Estrogen plus progestin and the incidence of dementia and mild cognitive impairment in postmenopausal women: The Women's Health Initiative Memory Study: a randomized controlled trial. JAMA 2003; 289(20): 2651–62.

15. Resnick SM, Henderson VW. Hormone therapy and risk of Alzheimer disease: a critical time. JAMA 2002; 288: 2170–2.

16. Feldman H, Jacova C. Primary prevention and delay of onset of AD/dementia. Can J Neurol Sci 2007 in press.

17. Roher AE, Esch C, Rahman A et al. Atherosclerosis of cerebral arteries in Alzheimer disease. Stroke 2001; 35(Suppl 1): 2623–7.

18. Forette F, Seux ML, Staessen JA et al. The prevention of dementia with antihypertensive treatment: new evidence from the Systolic Hypertension in Europe (Syst-Eur) study. Arch Intern Med 2002; 162(18): 2046–52.

19. Bosch J, Yusuf S, Pogue J et al. Use of ramipril in preventing stroke: double blind randomised trial. British Medical Journal 2002; 324(7339): 699–702.

20. Tzourio C, Anderson C, Chapman N et al. Effects of blood pressure lowering with perindopril and indapamide therapy on dementia and cognitive decline in patients with cerebrovascular disease. Arch Intern Med 2003; 163(9): 1069–75.

21. Skoog I, Lithell H, Hansson L et al. Effect of baseline cognitive function and antihypertensive treatment on cognitive and cardiovascular outcomes: study on cognition and prognosis in the elderly (SCOPE). Am J Hypertens 2005; 18(8): 1052–59.

22. Snowdon DA, Greiner LH, Mortimer JA et al. Brain infarction and the clinical expression of Alzheimer disease: the nun study. JAMA 1997; 277: 813–17.

23. Watson GS, Cholerton BA, Reger MA et al. Preserved cognition in patients with early Alzheimer disease and amnestic mild cognitive impairment during treatment with rosiglitazone: a preliminary study. Am J Geriatr Psychiatry 2005; 13(11): 950–8.

24. Collins R, Armitage J, Parish S, Sleigh P, Peto R. MRC/BHF Heart Protection Study of cholesterol-lowering with simvastatin in 5963 people with diabetes: a randomised placebo-controlled trial. Lancet 2003; 361(9374): 2005–16.

25. Shepherd J, Blauw GJ, Murphy MB et al. Pravastatin in elderly individuals at risk of vascular disease (PROSPER): a randomised controlled trial. Lancet 2002; 360(9346): 1623–30.

26. Wolozin B. A fluid connection: cholesterol and Abeta. Proc Natl Acad Sci USA 2001; 98(10), 5371–73.

27. Morris MC, Evans DA, Bienias JL et al. Dietary fats and the risk of incident Alzheimer disease. Arch Neurol 2003; 60(2): 194–200.

28. Lim GP, Calon F, Morihara T. A diet enriched with the omega-3 fatty acid docosahexaenoic acid reduces amyloid burden in an aged Alzheimer mouse model. J Neurosci 2005; 25(12): 3032–40.

29. Barberger-Gateau P, Letenneur L, Deschamps V. Fish, meat, and risk of dementia: cohort study. BMJ 2002; 325(7370): 932–3.

30. Whitmer RA, Gunderson EP, Barrett-Connor E, Quesenberry CP Jr, Yaffe K. Obesity in middle age and future risk of dementia: a 27 year longitudinal population based study. BMJ 2005; 330(7504): 1360.

31. Mattson MP. Existing data suggest that Alzheimer's disease is preventable. Ann NY Acad Sci 2000; 924: 153–9.

32. Stewart R, Masaki K, Xue QL et al. A 32-year prospective study of change in body weight and incident dementia: the Honolulu–Asia Aging Study. Arch Neurol 2005; 62(1): 55–60.

33. Tang MX, Jacobs D, Stern Y et al. Effect of oestrogen during menopause on risk and age at onset of Alzheimer's disease. Lancet 1996; 348: 429–32.

34. Hogervorst E, Yaffe K, Richards M, Huppert F. Hormone replacement therapy for cognitive function in postmenopausal women. Cochrane Database. Syst Rev 2002; (3): CD003122.

35. Shumaker SA, Legault C, Kuller L et al. Conjugated equine estrogens and incidence of probable dementia and mild cognitive impairment in postmenopausal women: Women's Health Initiative Memory Study. JAMA 2004; 291(24): 2947–58.

36. Yaffe K, Krueger K, Cummings SR et al. Effect of raloxifene on prevention of dementia and cognitive impairment in older women: the Multiple Outcomes of Raloxifene Evaluation (MORE) randomized trial. Am J Psychiatry 2005; 162(4), 683–690.

37. Etminan M, Gil S, Samii A. Effect of non-steroidal anti-inflammatory drugs on risk of Alzheimer's disease: systematic review and meta-analysis of observational studies. BMJ 2003; 327(7407): 128.

38. In't Veld VB, Ruitenberg A, Hofman A et al. Nonsteroidal antiinflammatory drugs and the risk of Alzheimer's disease. N Engl J Med 2001; 345(21): 1515–21.

39. Woodward M. Non AChEI treatment for AD: anti-inflammatory drugs. In Ritchie C, Ames D, Masters C, Cummings J, Eds. Therapeutic Strategies in Dementia. Oxford, UK: Clinical Publishing 2006.

40. Boyles, S. Naproxen may increase risk of heart disease. http://www.medscape.com/viewarticle/496403, accessed January 2006.

41. Petersen RC, Thomas RG, Grundman M et al. Vitamin E and donepezil for the treatment of mild cognitive impairment. N Engl J Med 2005; 352(23): 2379–88.

42. Feldman HH, Ferris S, Winblad-B et al. Effect of rivastigmine on delay to diagnosis of Alzheimer's disease from mild cognitive impairment: the InDDEx study. Lancet Neurology 2007: 6(6): 501–12.

43. Winblad B, Gauthier S, Scinto L et al; The GAL-INT-11/18 Study Group. Safety and efficacy of galantamine in subjects with mild cognitive impairment. Neurology 2008 Mar 5 [Epub ahead of print].

44. Wang HX, Wahlin A, Basun H et al. Vitamin B(12) and folate in relation to the development of Alzheimer's disease. Neurology 2001; 56(9): 1188–94.

45. Hogervorst E, Ribeiro HM, Molyneux A, Budge M, Smith AD. Plasma homocysteine levels, cerebrovascular risk factors, and cerebral white matter changes (leukoaraiosis) in patients with Alzheimer disease. Arch Neurol 2002; 59(5): 787–93.

46. Hassan A, Hunt BJ, O'Sullivan M et al. Homocysteine is a risk factor for cerebral small vessel disease, acting via endothelial dysfunction. Brain 2004; 127(Pt 1): 212–19.

47. Durga J, van Boxtel MP, Schouten EG et al. Effect of 3-year folic acid supplementation on cognitive function in older adults in the FACIT trial: a randomised, double blind, controlled trial. Lancet 2007; 369(9557); 208–16.

48. Engelhart J, Geerlings I, Ruiteberg A et al. Dietary intake of antioxidants and risk of Alzheimer disease. JAMA 2002; 287(24): 3223–9.

49. Morris MC, Evans DA, Bienias JL et al. Dietary intake of antioxidant nutrients and the risk of incident Alzheimer disease in a biracial community study. JAMA 2002; 287(24): 3230–7.

50. Miller ER, III, Pastor-Barriuso R, Dalal D et al. Meta-analysis: high-dosage vitamin E supplementation may increase all-cause mortality. Ann Intern Med 2005; 142(1): 37–46.

51. Scarmeas N, Levy G, Tang MX, Manly J, Stern Y. Influence of leisure activity on the incidence of Alzheimer's disease. Neurology 2001; 57(12): 2236–42.

52. Verghese J, Lipton RB, Katz MJ et al. Leisure activities and the risk of dementia in the elderly. N Engl J Med 2003; 348(25): 2508–16.

53. Kramer AF, Hahn S, Cohen NJ et al. Ageing, fitness and neurocognitive function. Nature 1999; 400(6743): 418–19.

54. Cahn-Weiner DA, Malloy DF, Rebok GW, Ott BR. Results of a randomized controlled study of memory training for mildly impaired Alzheimer's disease patients. Appl Neuropsychol 2003; 10(4): 215–23.

55. Davis RN, Massman PJ. Doody RS. Cognitive intervention in Alzheimer's disease: randomized placebo-controlled study. Alzheimer Dis Assoc Disord 2001; 15(1): 1–9.

56. Yaffe K, Barnes D, Nevitt M, Lui LY, Covinsky K. A prospective study of physical activity and cognitive decline in elderly women: women who walk. Arch Intern Med 2001; 161(14): 1703–8.

57. Weuve J, Kang JH, Manson JE et al. Physical activity, including walking, and cognitive function in older women. JAMA 2004; 292(12): 1454–61.

58. Molloy DW, Richardson LD, Crilly RG. The effects of a three-month exercise programme on neuropsychological function in elderly institutionalized women: a randomized controlled trial. Age Ageing 1988; 17(5): 303–10.

59. Emery CF, Schein RL, Hauck ER, MacIntyre NR. Psychological and cognitive outcomes of a randomized trial of exercise among patients with chronic obstructive pulmonary disease. Health Psychol 1998; 17(3): 232–40.

60. Lindsay J, Laurin D, Verreault R et al. Risk factors for Alzheimer's disease: a prospective analysis from the Canadian Study of Health and Aging. Am J Epidemiol 2002; 156: (5) 445–53.

61. Wilson RS, Mendes De Leon CF et al. Participation in cognitively stimulating activities and risk of incident Alzheimer disease. JAMA 2002; 287: 742–748.

62. Almeida OP, Hulse GK, Lawrence D, Flicker L. Smoking as a risk factor for Alzheimer's disease: contrasting evidence from a systematic review of case-control and cohort studies. Addiction 2000; 97(1): 15–28.

63. Ruitenberg A, van Swieten JC, Witteman JC et al. Alcohol consumption and risk of dementia: the Rotterdam Study. Lancet 2002; 359(9303): 281–6.

64. Mukamal KJ, Kuller LH, Fitzpatrick AL et al. Prospective study of alcohol consumption and risk of dementia in older adults. JAMA 2003; 289(11): 1405–13.

65. Doll R. Review: Alzheimer's disease and environmental aluminium. Age Ageing 1993; 22(2): 138–53.

66. Sobel E, Dunn M, Davanipour Z et al. Elevated risk of Alzheimer's disease among workers with likely electro-magnetic field exposure. Neurology 1996; 47: 1477–81.

67. Savitz DA, Checkoway H, Loomis DP. Magnetic field exposure and neurodegenerative disease mortality among electric utility workers. Epidemiology 1998; 9(4): 398–404.

68. Plassman B, Havlik R, Steffens D et al. Documented head injury in early adulthood and risk of Alzheimer's disease and other dementias. Neurology 2000; 55: 1158–66.

69. Mehta KM, Ott A, Kalmijn S et al Head trauma and risk of dementia and Alzheimer's disease: The Rotterdam Study. Neurology 1999; 53: 1959–62.

70. Fleminger S, Oliver DL, Lovestone S et al. (2003). Head injury as a risk factor for Alzheimer's disease: the evidence 10 years on; a partial replication. J Neurol Neurosurg Psychiatry 74(7): 857–62.

71. Launer LJ, Andersen K, Dewey ME et al. Rates and risk factors for dementia and Alzheimer's disease: results from EURODEM pooled analyses. EURODEM Incidence Research Group and Work Groups. European Studies of Dementia. Neurology 1999; 52: 78–84.

72. Karp A, Kareholt I, Qiu C et al. Relation of education and occupation-based socioeconomic status to incident Alzheimer's disease. Am J Epidemiol 2004; 159(2): 175–83.

73. Lee S, Kawachi I, Berkman LF, Grodstein F. Education, other socioeconomic indicators, and cognitive function. Am J Epidemiol 2003; 157(8): 712–20.

74. Smyth KA, Fritsch T, Cook TB, McClendon MJ et al. Worker functions and traits associated with occupations and the development of AD. Neurology 2004; 63(3): 498–503.

75. Helmer C, Letenneur L, Rouch I et al. Occupation during life and risk of dementia in French elderly community residents. J Neurol Neurosurg Psychiatry 2001; 71(3): 303–9.

76. US Alzheimer's Association. Maintain Your Brain. http://www.alz.org/maintainyourbrain/overview.asp, accessed 9: January 2006.

77. Centers for Disease Control and Prevention (1999). Decline in deaths from heart disease and stroke - United States, 1900-1999. JAMA 282(8): 724–6.

CHAPTER 7

Treatment of Alzheimer's disease
Najeeb Qadi, Michele Assaly, and Philip E Lee

INTRODUCTION

Alzheimer's disease (AD) is an illness that is set to create one of the world's largest socioeconomic healthcare burdens in the coming decades. This underscores the urgency of seeking effective therapeutic interventions for patients with AD. Current therapeutic approaches for AD have been developed to alleviate its symptoms and to modify its disease course.

SYMPTOMATIC TREATMENTS

Target symptoms

Symptomatic treatment is directed at the cognitive, behavioral, and functional disability in AD. It is also considered from a global or more holistic view. As symptoms emerge across the disease spectrum, the therapeutic targets do change. There are currently two licensed symptomatic treatments for AD, acetylcholinesterase inhibitors (ChEIs) and the uncompetitive NMDA receptor antagonist, memantine.

The ChEIs received regulatory approval by the Food and Drug Administration (FDA) and European agencies between 1993 and 2002 for mild to moderately severe AD. Recently, between 2002 and 2006, memantine was approved in the US and most countries worldwide. It has been licensed for the treatment of moderate to severe AD.

Figure 7.1 provides a schematic overview of the symptoms of AD from a mild cognitive impairment (MCI) stage through to profound AD. Individuals with MCI have cognitive decline, most often in the memory domain,

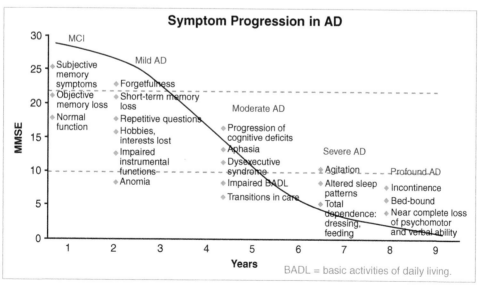

Figure 7.1   Symptom progression in Alzheimer's disease. MMSE = Mini-Mental State Examination; MCI = mild cognitive impairment; BADL = basic activities of daily living. Modified with permission from Feldman et al. The staging and assessment of moderate to severe Alzheimer disease. Neurology 2005; 65: S10–17.[2]

greater than that expected for an individual's age and education level, but that does not interfere significantly with activities of daily life.[1] In transition to mild AD, patients develop more apparent deficits in cognition that typically evolve from a core episodic memory impairment to other associative cortical regions, with resultant impairments in executive function, language, visuospatial domain, apraxia, and agnosia.[2] There is impairment in social functioning and loss of instrumental activities of daily living (IADL). There appears to be a transition point between the mild and moderate stage that has been suggested to occur at MMSE 16.[3] This transition represents a point where the illness becomes increasingly challenging and distressing to manage as functional decline crosses from instrumental to basic ADL. Psychobehavioral symptoms and cognitive losses also increase in moderately severe AD (MSAD). In MSAD, both short- and long-term memory systems fail, the ability to problem solve declines, and aphasia advances to a point at which communication abilities become marginal. The MSAD stages are accompanied by an increasing burden on caregivers, who also record increased levels of depressive symptoms.[4] In the severe stage of AD, patients lose awareness of all recent events. They are totally dependent for their basic activities of daily living. Agitation and aggression can be particularly problematic as are changes in sleep and circadian cycles. Severe AD transitions into the profound stage with clinical phenomenology well characterized by the Global Deterioration Scale (GDS)[5] stage 7. In this stage, patients are incontinent with near-complete loss of verbal ability and psychomotor skills. They are also largely bedbound.

Evaluating symptoms of AD

Cognition

Within clinical trials, the Alzheimer's Disease Assessment Scale–Cognitive Subscale (ADAS-cog)[6] has been most often used to measure cognitive change in mild to moderate AD. It is composed of 11 cognitive items that include spoken language ability, comprehension of spoken language, recall of test instructions, word-finding difficulty in spontaneous speech, following commands, naming objects and fingers, constructional praxis, ideational praxis, orientation, word-recall task, and word recognition task. The scale ranges between 0 and 70, with higher scores indicating greater impairment. ChEIs have consistently demonstrated a significant benefit on this measure compared to placebo in 6 month trials. The treatment effect size of ChEIs on average has been 2.7 points (95% confidence interval (CI) 2.3-3.0).[7] On average this corresponds to the naturalistic rate of decline in 6 months of disease at this mild to moderate stage.

The most common cognitive assessment measure in moderate to severe AD is the Severe Impairment Battery (SIB).[8] It takes into account the specific cognitive deficits associated with advanced AD. It includes more simplified measures, including some one-step commands that are presented in conjunction with gestural cues. The six major subscales probe attention, orientation, memory, language, visuospatial ability, and construction. In addition, there are also brief evaluations of praxis, social interaction, and orienting to name. Scale ranges from 0 to 100, with higher scores being better. In trials of memantine, the mean benefit in favor of memantine compared to placebo has been 2.97 points (95% CI 1.68-4.26).[9]

Global assessment

To meet regulatory specifications for approval of symptomatic drug treatments for AD, global clinical evaluations are also required. Instruments such as the Clinician's Interview-Based Impression of Change scale (CIBIC-Plus)[10] have been validated for such assessments. The CIBIC-Plus provides a global rating of patient function in four areas, general, cognitive, behavior, and activities of daily living. Information is obtained from the caregiver and patient. Patients are then rated on global severity at baseline and subsequent assessments on the 7-point Likert scale, where 1 indicates marked improvement and 7 marked worsening, with smaller changes in between. In the ChEI trials, when the CIBIC-Plus scale was dichotomized counting those showing no change or decline against those showing improvement and analyzed using the odds ratio (OR), benefits were associated with cholinesterase inhibitors (ChEIs) compared with placebo, with OR 1.56 (95% CI 1.32–1.85). When patients showing decline were dichotomized against patients showing improvement or no change, benefits associated with a ChEI compared with placebo were OR 1.84 (95% CI 1.47–2.30).[7] The memantine trials have also demonstrated a benefit of 0.28 points (95% CI 0.15–0.41) in favor of this medication compared to placebo.[9]

Neuropsychiatric symptoms

Neuropsychiatric symptoms (NPS) are particularly important as they emerge during the different stages of the disease. NPS progress over the course of the illness in parallel with cognitive decline. The severity of symptoms may correlate with the stage of dementia; however, they do vary considerably between patients. Apathy tends to be the most frequent NPS throughout AD. It is followed by agitation, anxiety, dysphoria, and aberrant motor behavior (Figure 7.2)[11].

The most widely used instrument to evaluate NPS is the Neuropsychiatric Inventory (NPI).[13] The NPI involves a semi-structured interview with a caregiver of a patient with dementia, in which the caregiver is asked to rate the frequency (0–4) and severity (0–3) of 12 NPS over the past 4 weeks. The 12 symptoms are: apathy, irritability/lability, dysphoria, delusions, hallucinations, euphoria, anxiety, agitation/aggression, disinhibition, aberrant motor activity, sleep disruption, and eating problems. The maximum score for each subscale is 12 (representing the frequency 3 severity score for each scale), where higher scores reflect greater impairment. The NPI total score is the sum of the subscale scores. ChEIs have demonstrated a benefit on the total NPI scores compared to placebo in 6 month trials, with a mean difference of 2.44 points (CI 4.12--0.76).[7] Memantine has also had a significant benefit on NPI total scores of 2.76 points (CI 0.88–4.63).[9]

Other scales, including the Behave AD Scale, Cornell Scale for Depression in Dementia, and Cohen-Mansfield Agitation Inventory, have all been used to capture the wide range of NPS.

Functional disability

For functional assessment, a variety of scales have been developed. The Disability Assessment for Dementia (DAD),[14] one of the more frequently used functional disability scales, employs a caregiver interview to address 40 items of ADL, 17 related to basic self-care and 23 to instrumental activities of daily living. ChEIs have shown benefit compared with placebo after 6 months or more of treatment, with a mean difference of 4.39 points (95% CI 1.96–6.81).[7] The Progressive Deterioration Scale (PDS)[15] is a 29-item caregiver assessment that is scored from 0 (greatest impairment) to 100. Again, ChEIs have shown benefit compared with placebo, with a mean difference of 2.40 points (95% CI 1.55–3.37).[7] The Alzheimer's Disease Cooperative Study-Activities of Daily Living (ADCS-ADL)[16] has also been used extensively within trials. The 23-item ADCS-ADL23 has 78 points, while the 19 item ADCS-ADLsev19 has 54 points, with higher number signifying greater impairment. In memantine trials, there was a significant benefit on the ADCS-ADLsev19 scale in favour of memantine, of 1.27 points (CI 0.44–2.09).[9]

Cholinesterase inhibitors

In the late 1970s, neurochemical deficits in the cholinergic system were first identified. It was appreciated that there was degeneration of the basal forebrain, particularly in the archipelago of cholinergic neurons of the substantia innominata, nucleus basalis of Meynert, and septal

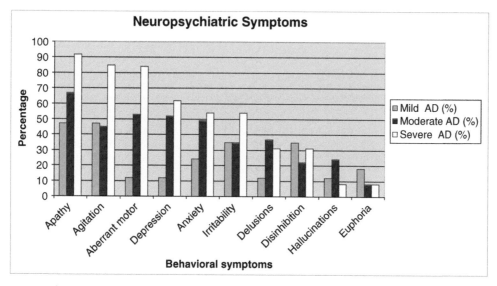

Figure 7.2 Neuropsychiatric symptoms in AD. Adapted with permission from Mega et al. The spectrum of behavioral changes in Alzheimer's disease. Neurology 1996; 46(1): 130–5[11] and Gauthier et al. Donepezil MSAD Study Investigators Group. Efficacy of donepezil on behavioral symptoms in patients with moderate to severe Alzheimer's disease. Int Psychogeriatrics 2002; 14(4): 389–404.[12]

nuclei.[17] ChEIs augment cholinergic levels and represent an accessible therapeutic direction.

Pharmacology (see Figure 7.3)

Physostigmine was the first ChEI tried in AD in 1979 with some symptomatic efficacy.[19] However, it did not present a favorable benefit-risk ratio given that acetylcholinesterase inhibition was limited, its selectivity was poor, and its penetration through the blood-brain barrier insufficient. These pioneering studies stimulated the successful development of the next generation of ChEIs, with markedly improved pharmacokinetic and pharmacodynamic profiles. Currently, four ChEIs (Tacrine, Donepezil, Rivastigmine, and Galantamine) are approved in most countries worldwide. In 1993, tacrine was the first ChEI approved for the treatment of AD. Its efficacy was demonstrated in trials of up to 6 months in patients with mild-to-moderate AD.[20]

As the first approved treatment it did reach some widespread use. However, its hepatic toxicity, its need for multiple daily doses, and the subsequent availability of better tolerated ChEIs led to its current status where it is rarely, if ever, prescribed.

In 1996, donepezil was the second ChEI that was approved for AD treatment. It is a piperidine derivative that non-competitively and reversibly blocks acetylcholinesterase. It is highly selective for acetylcholinesterase and is transported by binding to plasma proteins.[21,22]

Rivastigmine received its endorsement from the FDA in 2000. It is a slow, reversible dual inhibitor of both acetyl- and butyrylcholinesterase. It has only a very low capacity to bind to plasma proteins and is hydrolyzed intravascularly.[21,22] In 2007, rivastigmine received regulatory approval for a transdermal formulation that showed similar efficacy to highest oral doses within a large clinical trial, with three times fewer reports of nausea and vomiting.[23]

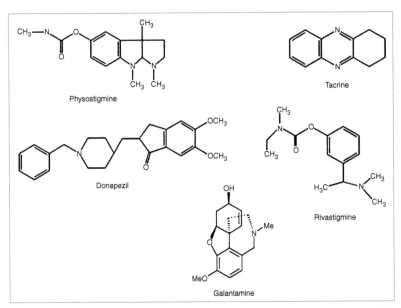

Figure 7.3 Chemical structure of AChEIs. Reproduced with permission from [18] and http://www.psycho pha rmacology.net/galantamine/ galan tam ine.jpg.

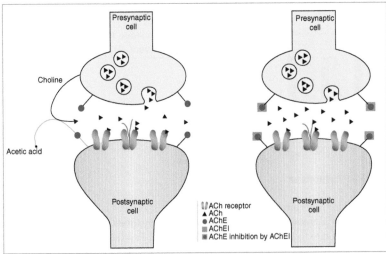

Figure 7.4 Mechanism of action of AChEIs. The neurotransmitter acetylcholine (ACh) is released from presynaptic vesicles into the synaptic cleft. ACh can bind to postsynaptic ACh receptors, activating them and causing an influx of Na^+ into the cell and an efflux of K^+ out of the cell. Termination of this synaptic activity is accomplished by the breakdown of ACh in the synaptic cleft to acetic acid and choline via the degrading enzyme acetylcholinesterase (AChE). Blocking the breakdown of ACh with acetylcholinesterase inhibitors (AChEIs) increases the amount of ACh available to activate postsynaptic receptors. Reproduced with permission from[24].

Galantamine, the fourth ChEI, received approval by the FDA in 2001. Galantamine is a selective reversible ChEI and acts as a positive allosteric ligand at nicotinic acetylcholine receptors, increasing the presynaptic release of acetylcholine and prolonging post-synaptic neurotransmission[21,22] (see Figure 7.4).

As demonstrated in Figures 7.5–7.7, the randomized clinical trials (RCTs) of ChEIs have demonstrated benefits in cognitive functioning, activities of daily living, and behavior for individuals with mild-to-moderately severe AD.[7]

The optimal duration of treatment with ChEIs is not fully resolved. Efficacy has been demonstrated for most

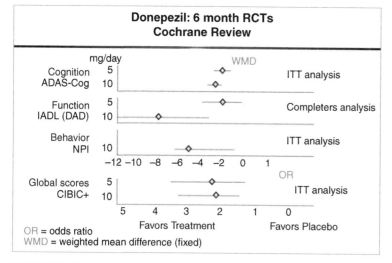

Figure 7.5 Effect of donepezil on different measures. Adapted with permission from Birks J. Cholinesterase inhibitors for Alzheimer's disease. Cochrane Database Syst Rev 2006; (1): CD005593.

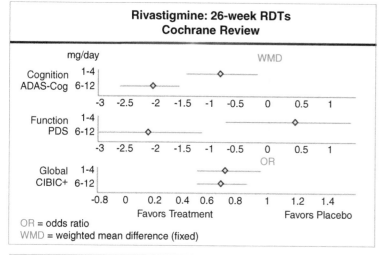

Figure 7.6 Effect of rivastigmine on different measures. Adapted with permission from Birks J. Cholinesterase inhibitors for Alzheimer's disease. Cochrane Database Syst Rev 2006; (1): CD005593.

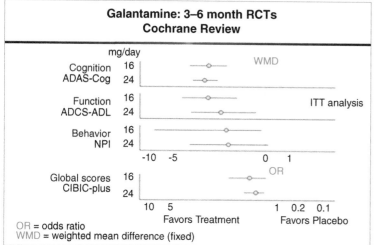

Figure 7.7 Effect of galantamine on several different measures. Adapted with permission from Birks J. Cholinesterase inhibitors for Alzheimer's disease. Cochrane Database Syst Rev 2006; (1): CD005593.

RCTs within 6–12 months, 24–26 as well as in a few placebo controlled trials of ≥ 1 year.[28,29] The open-label extension trials of some of the short-duration, double-blind RCTs have suggested the benefits of treatment may extend up to 5 years.[30,31] These uncontrolled open-label extension studies likely have significant survivor bias, leaving uncertainty over the duration of benefit of ChEIs.

The concurrent administration of more than one ChEI at a time is not recommended, as there have been no safety studies conducted and the likelihood of induced excessive cholinergic side-effects is higher. The indications for switching from one ChEI to another include unmanageable side-effects or unmitigated cognitive decline after a treatment trial lasting at least 6 months.[32]

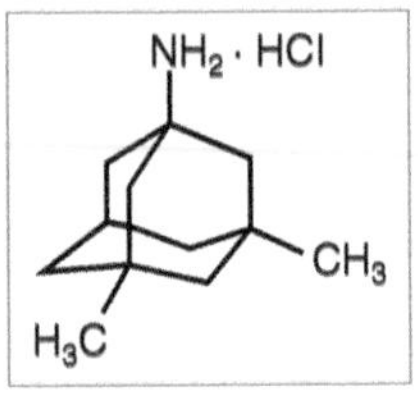

Adverse events reported in the trials include a range of cholinergic side-effects such as abdominal pain, anorexia, nausea, vomiting, diarrhea, weight loss, abnormal dreams, dizziness, fatigue, headache, insomnia, muscle cramp, peripheral edema, syncope, tremor, vertigo, and asthenia. The cholinergic side effect profile varies across the agents, though they have not concurrently been tested within a clinical trial for direct side by side comparison. Adverse events often occur during the initiation of treatment and they are generally lower during maintenance therapy. The general approach to ChEIs is to initially introduce agents at their lowest dosage and, thereafter, slowly increase the dosage at monthly intervals to the maximum and best tolerated dose. Administering the medications with meals may limit gastrointestinal side-effects.

There has been some public debate around the cost effectiveness of the ChEIs. According to the recent recommendations by the National Institute for Health and Clinical Excellence (NICE) in the UK, cholinesterase inhibitors were supported for the treatment of patients with AD with MMSE scores of 10–20,[33] while other paying agencies have different coverage formulas. The dosage and titration of these medications are presented in Table 7.1.

Memantine (20 mg daily)
Low to mod affinity voltage dependent,
uncompetitive NMDA receptor antagonist

Figure 7.8 Chemical structure of memantine. Reproduced with permission from http://www.rxlist.com/cgi/generic3/namenda.htm.

Table 7.1 Dosage, frequency, and titration of symptomatic AD treatment

Pharmacologic agent	Mechanism of action	Route	Starting dose	Titration schedule	Maximum dose	Metabolism
Donepezil	ChEI	Per os by tablets or by orally disintegrating tablets	5 mg once daily	Increase by 5 mg after 4–6 weeks as tolerated	10 mg once daily	Hepatic CYP2D6, CYP3A4
Rivastigmine	ChEI and butyryl-cholinesterase inhibitor	per os by tablets	1.5 mg twice daily	Increase by 1.5 mg twice daily every 4–6 weeks as tolerated	6 mg twice daily	Renal clearance
Rivastigmine	ChEI and butyryl-cholinesterase inhibitor	Transdermal	4.6 mg/24 hours patch (5 cm²) once daily	Increase to 9.5 mg for 10 cm² patch daily after 4 weeks	9.5 mg/24 hours patch (10 cm²) once daily	Renal clearance
Galantamine	ChEI and nicotinic receptor modulator	Per os by capsule	8 mg extended release once daily	Increase by 8 mg every 4–6 weeks as tolerated	24 mg extended release once daily	Hepatic CYP2D6, CYP3A4
Memantine	Uncompetitive NMDA antagonist	Per os by tablet	5 mg once daily	Increase by 5 mg every week as tolerated	10 mg twice daily	Predominant renal clearance

Glutamate antagonists

Glutamatergic neurotransmission represents another neurochemical target in AD. Glutamate is the major excitatory neurotransmitter in the central nervous system and plays an important role both in long term potentiation and synaptic plasticity, which are considered to underlie learning and memory.[34] An increase in extracellular glutamate can also lead to excessive activation of N-methyl-D-aspartate (NMDA) receptors and consequently intracellular calcium accumulation, which can induce a cascade resulting in neuronal death by necrosis or apoptosis.[35]

Memantine is an uncompetitive, moderate-affinity, NMDA antagonist that protects neurons against glutamate-mediated excitotoxicity (Figures 7.8 and 7.9). As demonstrated in Figures 7.10a–d the RCTs of memantine have mostly demonstrated benefits in cognitive functioning, global functioning, activities of daily living, and behavior for individuals with moderate to severe AD.[36–38]

There has been one study reporting on the combination of memantine with donepezil. This study demonstrated significant cognitive and behavioral improvement on SIB and NPI for patients who were given memantine while being already on donepezil, in comparison with patients who were on donepezil and placebo.[38] (Figures 7.11a and b).

Pharmacology

The dosage and titration of memantine are presented in Table 7.1. It is a generally well tolerated medication. In pivotal registration trials, the most frequently reported side-effects of memantine were agitation, confusion, diarrhea, and flu-like symptoms. However, agitation was significantly more common with placebo than with memantine treatment.

According to NICE, memantine is not currently recommended as a treatment option for people with moderately severe or severe Alzheimer's disease except as part of clinical research studies,[33] while it has been more widely used in the US and other countries.

Other symptomatic management of neuropsychiatric symptoms

When NPS develop, the trigger factors and causes need to be looked into, as some may be treatable without specific pharmacology. Furthermore, a variety of

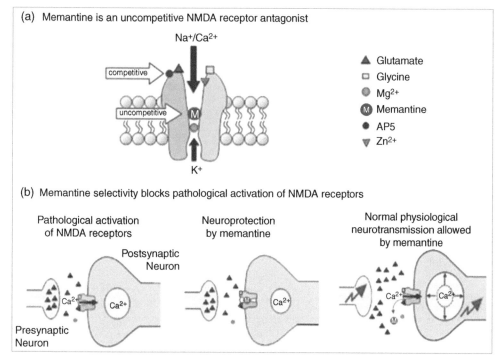

Figure 7.9 Memantine mechanism of action. (a) The glutamatergic NMDA receptor is activated when co-agonists glutamate and glycine bind to their respective subunits, and a concomitant positive change in membrane potential occurs to relieve the magnesium blockade of the channel pore. Memantine inhibits NMDA receptor activity by binding to a site other than that to which glutamate binds (uncompetitive antagonist). (b) It is believed that memantine selectively blocks pathologic activation of NMDA receptors yet exits the channel pore to allow normal physiologic neurotransmission under conditions of learning and memory formation. Reproduced with permission from Farlow MR. Geriatrics 2004; 59(6): 22–7.

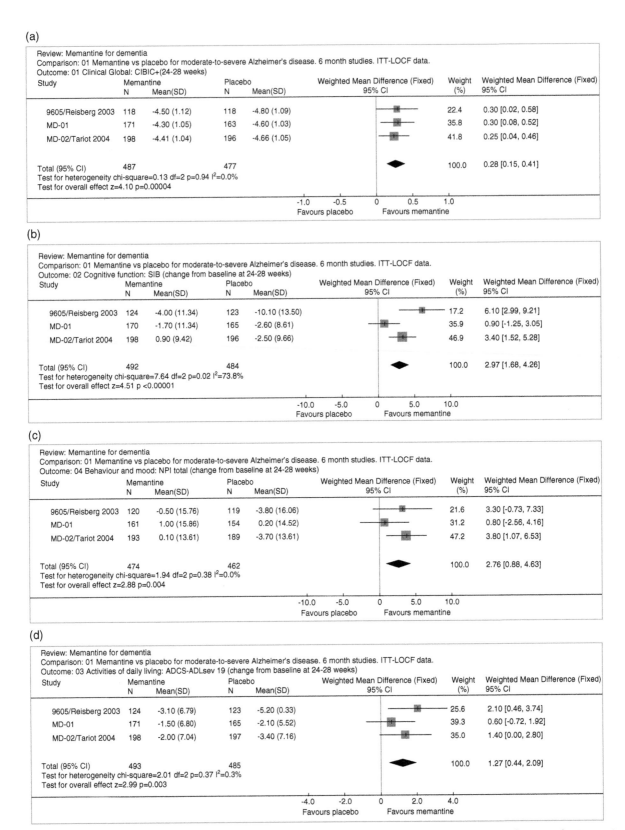

Figure 7.10 (a) Memantine effect on a global measure in AD. Reproduced with permission from McShane et al. Memantine for dementia. Cochrane Database Syst Rev 2006; (2): CD003154.[9] (b) Memantine effect on a cognitive measure in AD. Reproduced with permission from McShane et al. Memantine for dementia. Cochrane Database Syst Rev 2006; (2): CD003154.[9] (c) Memantine effect on a behavioral measure in AD. Reproduced with permission from McShane et al. Memantine for dementia. Cochrane Database Syst Rev 2006; (2): CD003154.[9] (d) Memantine effect on a functional measure in AD. Reproduced with permission from McShane et al. Memantine for dementia. Cochrane Database Syst Rev 2006; (2): CD003154.[9]

(a)

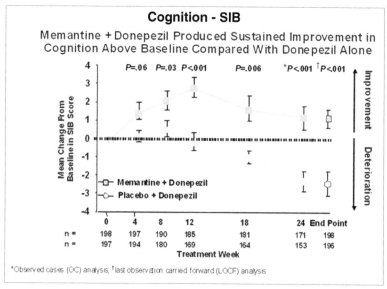
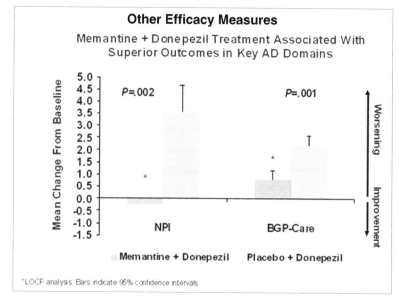

Figure 7.11 (a) Memantine + donepezil in a moderate-to severe AD study. Adapted with permission from Tariot et al. Memantine treatment in patients with moderate to severe Alzheimer disease already receiving donepezil: a randomized controlled trial. JAMA 2004; 291: 317–24. (b) Memantine + ChEI effect on behavioral and ADL measures in AD. Adapted with permission from Tariot et al. Memantine treatment in patients with moderate to severe Alzheimer disease already receiving donepezil: a randomized controlled trial. JAMA 2004; 291: 317–24.

non-pharmacologic interventions have been systematically studied for the treatment of behavioral disturbances in AD. Formal programs such as reality orientation, reminiscence therapy, and validation therapy have all been shown to have a positive effect, to some extent, on behavior, social interaction, well-being, and cognition.[39] Several therapies centering on sensory stimulation have been shown to be effective in reducing agitation and behavioral problems. Music therapy delivered via various methods has also been reported as an effective treatment. However, according to Cochrane Review, the methodologic quality and the reporting of the studies have been insufficient to draw any useful conclusions.[40] Beyond the use of non-pharmacologic

treatments, medications are often required, particularly for acute target symptoms.

Apathy

As the most prevalent NPS, apathy is particularly important and often underrecognized. It is commonly defined as a lack of interest, emotion, and motivation. Interventions, including behavioral techniques, which optimize functioning, initiate goal-directed behaviors, and increase involvement in pleasant activities, are useful. With regards to pharmacologic interventions there have been very few studies of any medications, but post-hoc analyses suggest that ChEIs may be effective in

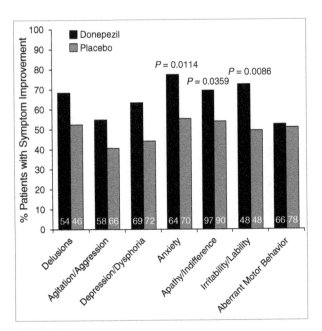

Figure 7.12 Symptom improvement* at week 24 LOCF in the most common symptoms present at baseline. *Improvement defined as patients who had a symptom at baseline, and a lower NPI item score at their final visit; percentages based on total number of patients who had the symptom at baseline, within each treatment group (numbers in bars). LOCF = last observation carried forward; NPI = Neuropsychiatric Inventory. Reproduced with permission[12].

the treatment of apathy as well as irritability and anxiety (see Figure 7.12).[12]

Depression

The presence of depression has been correlated with increased disability, impaired quality of life, and higher mortality. It can be observed in 20–40% of patients with AD.[41] There is reported greater cell loss in the locus ceruleus with reduced cortical serotonin reuptake sites in individuals with depressive symptoms, compared with those without such symptoms. Several clinical trials have addressed the treatment of depression in patients with AD, most of which have been inconclusive. Treatment should probably be reserved for patients with major depression. Selective serotonin-reuptake inhibitors (SSRIs) and tricyclic antidepressants (TCAs) have been used for treating depression, however the preferred choice is an SSRI.[42] TCAs are best avoided as they can increase cognitive and functional impairments in AD (see Table 7.2).

Psychosis and agitation

With regard to psychosis, non-pharmacologic interventions include the correction of visual and hearing impairments as well as improving lighting to reduce the risk of misinterpretations. For the pharmacologic treatment of psychotic symptoms such as delusions and hallucinations, antipsychotic medications, either typicals or atypicals, are commonly prescribed. Typical antipsychotics include chlorpromazine and haloperidol, medications that work by primarily blocking dopamine receptors in the brain. Sedation, extrapyramidal symptoms, and falls have been associated with the use of these antipsychotics. The atypical antipsychotic medications include quetiapine, clozapine, resperidone, olanzapine, ziprasidone, and aripiprazole. When a patient with dementia requires treatment with an antipsychotic agent for the management of psychosis or agitation, an atypical antipsychotic is preferable. They produce fewer side-effects such as parkinsonism and tardive dyskinesia than conventional neuroleptic drugs. However, there has been warning labeling regarding a potential association between the use of these atypical antipsychotic medications and cerebrovascular events as well as death.[44] In the face of these warnings, antipsychotic medications should be used as infrequently as possible and at the lowest doses possible to minimize adverse effects. Efforts should be made to taper the medication and discontinue it as soon as practically feasible.

Mood-stabilizing agents may also reduce behavioral disturbances in patients with AD. Agitation appeared to improve significantly in trials with carbamazepine.[45] Divalproex sodium has been studied for its effects on agitation, with mixed results. Patients with inadequate responses to antipsychotics may benefit from therapy with mood stabilizers or antidepressants alone or in combination with antipsychotic agents. There is still a clear need for improved symptomatic therapies to address the variety of other neuropsychiatric disturbances associated with disease.

DISEASE-MODIFYING THERAPEUTIC STRATEGIES

Enormous research attention is currently being directed at the strategies designed to modify AD pathogenesis. These approaches are directed at slowing or halting the progression of the disease. Though none are yet proven, it might be foreseen that such treatments are on the edge of potential breakthrough. If successful, they will be used in conjunction with existing symptomatic therapies (see Figure 7.13).

Table 7.2 Nine randomised, placebo-controlled trials that evaluated the efficacy of pharmacologic interventions in reducing depression among patients dementia

Summary of Evidence-Based Pharmacological Treatment for Depression in Dementia

Study type	n	Medication (daily dose)	Baseline pt. with dementia and depression (%)	Impact on depression	Impact on cognition	Impact on BPSD	Impact on functional status
6 week RCT (Myth et al. [1992]: Acta Psychiatr Scand 86[2]: 138–145)	149	Citalopram (30 mg max)	19.5%	+	NA	+	NA
12 week crossover RCT with 2 week washout (Petracca et al. [1996]: J Neuropsychiatry Clin Neurosci 8[3]: 270–275)	24	Clomipramine	100% (100 mg max)	+	–	NA	NS
8 week RCT (Reifler et al. [1989]: Am J Psychiatry 146[1]:45–49)	61	Imipramine (83 mg mean)	50%	+	NS	NS	NS
6 week RCT (Roth et al. [1995]: Br J Psychiatry 158[2]:149–157)	694	Moclobemide (400 mg max)	75%	+	NS	NA	NS
8 week RCT (Fuchs et al. [1993]: Pharmacopsychiatry 26[2]:37–41)	127	Maprotiline (75 mg max)	100%	+	NS	NA	NA
12 week RCT (Lyketeos et al. [2003]: Arch Gen/Psychiatry 60[7]: 737–746)	44	Sertraline (95 mg mean)	100%	+	NS	+	+
6 week RCT (Petracca et al. [2001]: Int Psychogentatr 13[2]:233–240)	41	Fluoxetine (40 mg max)	100%	NS	NS	NS	NS

(Continued)

Table 7.2 (Continued)

Summary of Evidence-Based Pharmacological Treatment for Depression in Dementia

Study type	n	Medication (daily dose)	Baseline pt. with dementia and depression (%)	Impact on depression	Impact on cognition	Impact on BPSD	Impact on functional status
8 week RCT (Magai et al. [2000]: Am J Geriatr Psychiatry 8[1]: 66–74)	31	Sertraline	100%	NS	NS	NS	NS
4 week RCT (Myth and Gettfrias [1990]: Br J Psychiatry 157: 894–901)	98	Citalopram (30 mg max)	All patients had dementia but only 10% had major depression	NS	NS	+	NA

+ = positive effect
− = negative effect

NS = no significant effect
NA = not available

RCT = randomized controlled trial
N = total number of subjects in the trial
BPSD = behavioral and psychological symptoms of dementia
Source: Boustri M (2004)

Reproduced with permission from Boustani M, Watson L. The interface of depression and dementia. Psychiatric Times 2004; XXI: Issue 3.[43]

Detailed discussion of the pathogenesis of AD can be found in Chapter 4 Pathophysiology of Alzheimer's disease. The following sections describe those disease-modifying approaches currently in development.

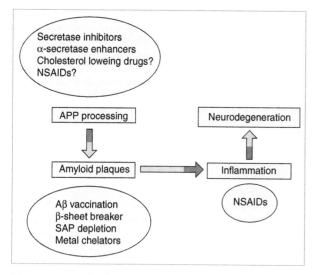

Figure 7.13 The figure summarizes the main hypothesized pathologic processes and the related therapeutic approaches in AD. NSAIDs = non-steroidal anti-inflammatory drugs; APP = amyloid precursor protein; SAP = serum amyloid P component. Reproduced with permission from [46].

Modulation of secretases

Beta (β) and gamma (γ) secretase inhibitors are being developed to reduce the neurotoxic amyloidogenic moieties including toxic oligomers and protofibrils. γ-Secretase seems to be more accessible as its inhibition appears to be possible without dangerous disturbance of other essential enzyme activity. Phase III clinical trials are being conducted for γ-secretase inhibitors and modulators. b-Secretase inhibition has been so far inaccessible and there are no current candidates in clinical trials.[47]

Aβ vaccination

In 1999, a potentially new avenue of AD therapy was developed through vaccination of transgenic APP mice (PDAPP) with fibrillar human Aβ42. In transgenic mice, overexpressing human APP and having increased Ab, vaccination of full length 1–42 almost completely prevented amyloid deposition after 11 months of continuous vaccination, with a significant delay of the progression of AD pathology (see Figure 7.14).[48] Subsequent studies in various AD mouse models confirmed the beneficial effects of this immunotherapy on behavioral and neuropathologic changes.

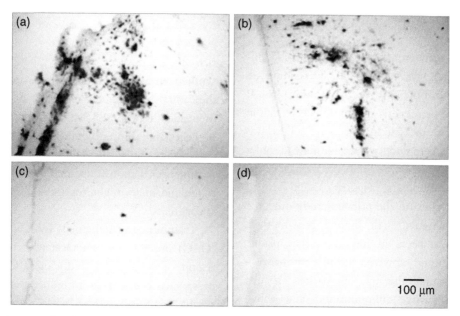

Figure 7.14 Reduction of Aβ burden in the entorhinal (EC) and retrosplenial (RSC) cortex of older PDAPP mice following Aβ injection. Aβ deposition in the RSC and EC cortices of 15-month-old PBS- (a, b) and Aβ42- (c, d) injected mice with Aβ burdens representative of the median values of their respective groups. Aβ deposition was greatly reduced in the RSC of Aβ42-injected mice compared with the PBS group (compare a and c). No Aβ was detected in the EC of Aβ42-injected mice (d), in contrast to the PBS group (b). Scale bar in (d) corresponds to all panels. Reproduced with permission from Schenk et al. Immunization with amyloid-beta attenuates Alzheimer-disease-like pathology in the PDAPP mouse. Nature 1999; 400(6740): 173–7.[48]

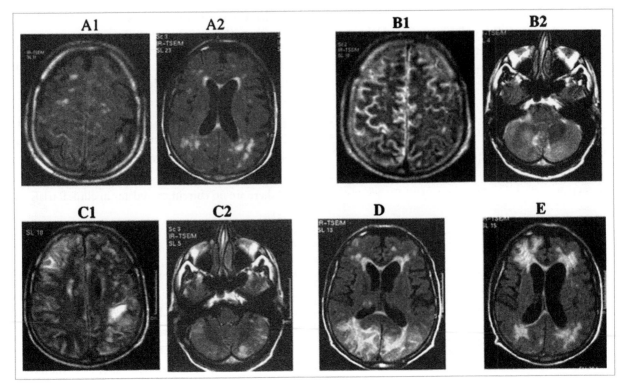

Figure 7.15 Serial brain MRI scans of patient with meningoencephalitis. Images performed 22 days (A1 and A2), 41 days (B1 and B2), 64 days (C1 and C2), 87 days (D), and 170 days (E) after immunization. (A) Presence of high signal intensities in the subcortical white matter and in the central sulcus (A1); numerous high signal intensities in the deep white matter (A2). (B) All sulci present an increased signal intensity that is related to the presence of protein in the CSF (B1); new lesions in the white matter of the right cerebellar peduncle (B2). (C) Worsening in the number and location of the lesions, now affecting the white matter and the gray matter of the cerebral (C1) and the cerebellar cortex (C2), while the lesions in the cerebellar peduncle have disappeared. (D) Extensive new lesions in the deep posterior white matter also affecting the adjacent cortex. (E) New lesions in the deep frontal white matter, while some lesions in the posterior white matter disappeared. Reproduced with permission from Orgogozo JM et al. Subacute meningoencephalitis in a subset of patients with AD after Abeta[42] immunization. Neurology 2003; 61(1): 46–54.[49]

Subsequent to these promising results, a phase I clinical trial of a human AD vaccine (AN-1792) was completed, followed by a phase II trial. In March 2002, this phase II trial was suspended after reports of meningoencephalitis in 6% of subjects, in the vaccination arm.[49] This was presumed to have been induced autoimmune disorder with activated T-lymphocytes and macrophages that caused severe inflammation (see Figures 7.15 and 7.16).

The clinical results on the primary study outcome measures were negative.[50] In limited post-mortem material, there has been an indication that plaque burden was significantly lowered through the neocortex.[51] Other immunotherapy approaches against amyloid involve passive immunization and active immunization with smaller amyloid fragments.

Amyloid antiaggregants

As Ab forms into protofibrils, they undergo a conformational change that causes an aggregation of a fibril rich β-pleated sheet. Short synthetic peptides, called synthetic mini-chaperones, which are homologous to the central hydrophobic region of Aβ, are in development and it is proposed that these peptides could disrupt β-sheet stabilization.[52] Clinical trials of antiaggregants as potential therapies for AD are entering into trials. A recent paper demonstrated that preventing oligomers in transgenic mice might represent a novel approach to antiaggregates.[53]

Tramiprosate (Alzhemed) is a glycos-amino-glycan (GAG) mimetic that interacts with the GAG-binding region of soluble Aβ, reducing fibrilization. Tramiprosate has been shown to reduce the accumulation of soluble and fibrillar Ab in transgenic mice.[54] A phase II study in individuals with mild-to-moderate AD demonstrated tolerability, safety, and brain penetration, as well as decreased CSF Aβ level.[55] A phase III trial is currently underway to determine its benefit in mild-to-moderate AD patients.

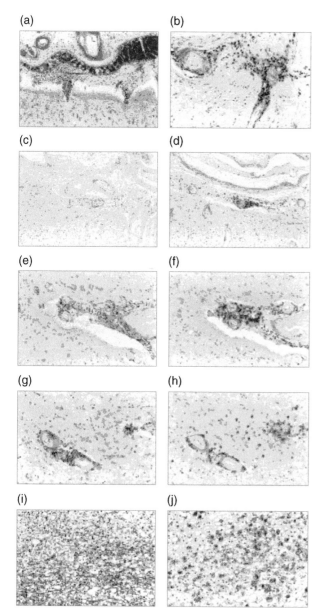

Figure 7.16 Meningoencephalitis and infiltration of cerebral white matter by macrophages. (a–h), Leptomeningeal infiltrate of lymphocytes stained with H&E (a) and immunostained with a T-lymphocyte antibody (CD3; b). No B-lymphocytes were detected (CD79a; c). (d–h), Area adjacent to (c) showing T-lymphocyte (CD3-positive) aggregation around meningeal blood vessels. Meningeal lymphocytes are predominantly CD8-negative (e) and CD4-positive (f). Lymphocytes within the cerebral neocortex are also predominantly CD8-negative (g) and CD4-positive (h). (i), Vacuolation and rarefaction of myelinated fibers in the cerebral white matter. (j), Infiltration of cerebral white matter by CD68-immunoreactive macrophages. Reproduced with permission from Nicoll et al. Neuropathology of human Alzheimer disease after immunization with amyloid-beta peptide: a case report. Nature Medicine 2003; 9(4): 448–52.[51]

Amyloid aggregation also requires its coupling with heavy ion metals, such as copper and zinc. Potentially, chelators of these ions could reduce aggregation. Clioquinol, an antiparasitic drug, has been found to be an effective metal chelator that can markedly reduce aggregated amyloid in transgenic mice.[56] A phase II randomized controlled trial (RCT) of clioquinol in patients with mild-to-moderate AD demonstrated some evidence of cognitive benefits with treatment and reduction of plasma Ab levels.[57] However, clioquinol is likely not the ideal drug, having been removed from the market many years ago, for myelo-optico-neuropathy. Alternative chelating agents to reduce amyloid accumulation without this toxicity are being pursued.

Intravenous immunoglobulin (IVIg) is a therapy that has been receiving current attention. It is a plasma product that is formed from pooled donor IgG antibodies. IVIg contains anti-Aβ antibodies which may augment the clearance of Ab.[58] Levels of anti-Ab antibodies are lower in AD patients compared to healthy individuals.[59] In preliminary AD clinical trials, IVIg had several positive effects including the lowering of soluble Ab and the stabilization of cognitive decline, with improved cognition in several patients.[60]

Antioxidants

Antioxidants have attracted attention as a potential therapy to reduce free radical damage resulting from increased oxidative stress. The principal antioxidant strategy that has been investigated has been treatment with alpha-tocopherol (vitamin E). The proposal that oxidative stress contributes to AD was the basis for including vitamin E 2000 IU daily in a multi-arm study of moderate-to-severe AD. In this study there was a significant delay in the time to the primary outcomes of death, institutionalization, loss of the ability to perform basic activities of daily living, or severe dementia.[61] However, a recent RCT using vitamin E in individuals with mild cognitive impairment for a period of 3 years showed no improvement with the usage of vitamin E.[62] Furthermore, a meta-analysis has demonstrated both increased cardiac side-effects in individuals taking large doses of vitamin E and increased mortality risk. These have effectively removed vitamin E as a therapeutic option (see Figure 7.17).[63]

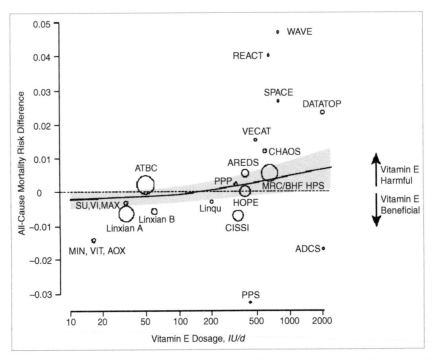

Figure 7.17   Effect of high and low doses of Vitamin E on mortality. The risk trend is the *solid curve* and its 95% confidence band is in the *shaded region*. Circled areas are proportional to the inverse of study variance in the analysis. ADCS = Alzheimer's Disease Cooperative Study; AREDS = Age-Related Eye Diseases Study; ATBC = Alpha-Tocopherol, Beta Carotene Cancer Prevention Study Group; CHAOS = Cambridge Heart Antioxidant Study; DATATOP = Deprenyl and Tocopherol Antioxidative Therapy of Parkinsonism; GISSI-Prevenzione = Gruppo Italiano per lo Studio della Sopravvivenza nell'Infarcto Miocardio Prevenzione; HOPE = Heart Outcomes Prevention Evaluation; MIN.VIT.AOX = The Geriatrie/MINéraux, VITamines, et AntiOXydants Network; MRC/BHF HPS = Medical Research Council/British Heart Foundation Heart Protection Study; PPP = Primary Prevention Project; PPS = Polyp Prevention Study; REACT = Roche European American Cataract Trial; SPACE = Secondary Prevention with Antioxidants of Cardiovascular disease in Endstage renal disease; SU.VI.MAX = SUpplementation en VItamines et Minéraux AntioXydants; VECAT = Vitamin E, Cataracts, and Age-Related Maculopathy; WAVE = Women's Angiographic Vitamin and Estrogen. Reproduced with permission from Miller et al. Meta-analysis: high-dosage vitamin E supplementation may increase all-cause mortality. Annals of Internal Medicine 2005;142(1): 37–46.[63]

Antibiotics

It has been hypothesized that antibiotics such as rifampicin and tetracycline have anti-amyloidogenic activity. Rifampicin may inhibit Aβ aggregation and its neurotoxicity through scavenging of free radicals. Tetracycline may be an antiaggregant as it seems able to disassemble amyloid aggregants *in vitro* and may therefore interfere with deposition of amyloid in AD. A recent RCT demonstrated that therapy with a combination of doxycycline and rifampin may have a therapeutic role in patients with mild to moderate AD.[64] Further confirmatory trials are needed.

Anti-inflammatory agents

The use of anti-inflammatory agents is based on the postulation that inflammation is centrally involved in the AD pathologic cascade. There has also been tantalizing epidemiological evidence that non-steroidal anti-inflammatory drugs (NSAID) use reduces AD risk. However, large trials of glucocorticoid therapy, hydroxychloroquine, and NSAIDs in the treatment of AD have so far been disappointing and their utility in disease modification has not been demonstrated.[65] Therefore, there is no evidence to support treatment with NSAIDs for AD.

Cholesterol-lowering agents

An important relationship between metabolism and transport of cholesterol and Ab has been recognized. Excess brain cholesterol has been associated with increased formation and deposition of Ab from amyloid precursor protein. High neuronal cholesterol may also

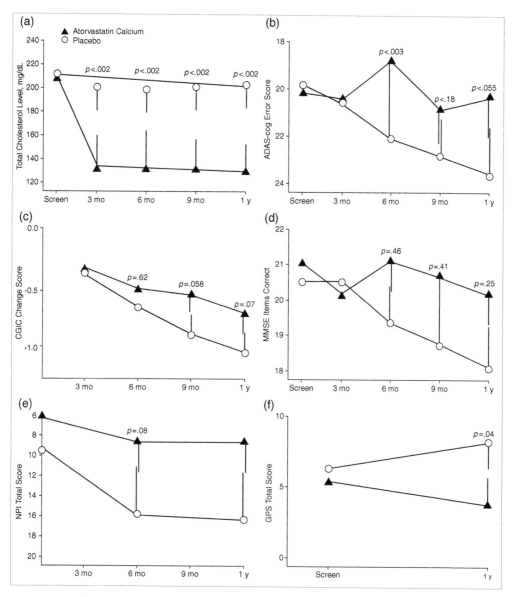

Figure 7.18 Atorvastatin effect on different scales. Reproduced with permission from Sparks DL et al. Atorvastatin for the treatment of mild to moderate Alzheimer disease: preliminary results. Archives of Neurology 2005; 62: 753–7.[67]

impair α-secretase and secondarily lead to increased Ab.[66] The utility of statins (HMG-CoA reductase inhibitors) is being investigated. In a recent pilot study of mild-to-moderate AD, there was a trend towards benefit with atorvastatin treatment at 12 months on cognitive, global, and behavioral outcomes[67] (Figure 7.18). A larger scale study is currently being undertaken in mild-to-moderate AD.

Neurotropic factors

Cerebrolysin (FPF-1070) is a preparation of amino acids and peptides derived from purified porcine brain proteins. It is postulated to exhibit neurotropic activity similar to nerve growth factor,[68] and may play a role in preserving cholinergic neurons.[69] In a transgenic mouse model of AD, administration of Cerebrolysin reduced the size of amyloid plaques, possibly by regulating amyloid precursor protein maturation and decreasing transport to sites of Ab protein production.[70] There has been some reported efficacy in randomized clinical trials performed in subjects with AD where the administration of intravenous administration of cerebrolysin demonstrated improvements on measures of cognition, global rating and activities of daily living.[71–74] Though cerebrolysin appeared to be well tolerated, it is still at a stage of research interest requiring further study to see if there is sufficient efficacy and safety to reach regulatory approval.

CONCLUSION

In the last hundred years, much has been elucidated in our understanding of the pathogenesis of the disease. Current treatments for patients with AD target the biochemical pathways that are associated with the disease. Current symptomatic treatments can ease disease burden by positively impacting cognition, function, and NPS. The development of interventions that can substantially delay the onset or modify the progression of AD is eagerly anticipated.

REFERENCES

1. Gauthier S, Reisberg B, Zaudig M et al. Mild cognitive impairment. Lancet 2006; 367(9518): 1262–70.

2. Feldman HH, Woodward M. The staging and assessment of moderate to severe Alzheimer disease. Neurology 2005; 65(Suppl 3): S10–S17.

3. Feldman H, Van BB, Kavanagh SM et al. Cognition, function, and caregiving time patterns in patients with mild-to-moderate Alzheimer's disease: a 12-month analysis. Alzheimer Dis Assoc Disord 2005; 19: 29–36.

4. Baumgarten M, Hanley JA, Infante-Rivard C et al. Health of family members caring for elderly persons with dementia. A longitudinal study. Ann Intern Med 1994; 120: 126–32.

5. Reisberg B, Ferris SH, de Leon MJ. The global deterioration scale for assessment of primary degenerative dementia. Am J Psychiatry 1982; 139: 1136.

6. Rosen WG, Mohs RC, Davis KL. A new rating scale for Alzheimer's disease. Am J Psychiatry 1984; 141: 1356–64.

7. Birks J. Cholinesterase inhibitors for Alzheimer's disease. Cochrane Database Syst Rev 2006; (1): CD005593.

8. Saxton J, McGonigle-Gibson KL, Swihart AA et al. Assessment of the severely impaired patient: description and validation of a new neuropsychological test battery. Psychol Assess 1990; 2: 298–303.

9. McShane R, Areosa Sastre A, Minakaran N. Memantine for dementia. Cochrane Database Syst Rev 2006; (2): CD003154.

10. Schneider LS, Olin JT, Doody RS et al. Validity and reliability of the Alzheimer's Disease Cooperative Study - Clinical Global Impression of Change. Alzheimer Dis Assoc Disord 1997; 11 (Suppl 2): S22–S32.

11. Mega MS, Cummings JL, Fiorello T et al. The spectrum of behavioral changes in Alzheimer's disease. Neurology 1996; 46(1): 130–5.

12. Gauthier S, Feldman H, Hecker J et al. Donepezil MSAD Study Investigators Group. Efficacy of donepezil on behavioral symptoms in patients with moderate to severe Alzheimer's disease. Int Psychogeriatr 2002; 14(4): 389–404.

13. Cummings JL, Mega M, Gray K et al. The Neuropsychiatric Inventory. Neurology 1994; 44: 2308–14.

14. Gelinas I, Gauthier L, McIntyre M et al. Development of a functional measure for persons with Alzheimer's disease: the Disability Assessment for Dementia. Am J Occup Ther 1999; 53: 471–81.

15. DeJong R, Osterlund OW, Roy GW. Measurement of quality-of-life changes in patients with Alzheimer's disease. Clin Ther 1989; 11(4): 545–54.

16. Galasko D, Bennett D, Sano M et al. An inventory to assess activities of daily living for clinical trials in Alzheimer's disease. The Alzheimer's Disease Cooperative Study. Alzheimer Dis Assoc Disord 1997; 11(Suppl 2): S33–S39.

17. Whitehouse PJ, Price DL, Clark AW et al. Alzheimer disease: evidence for selective loss of cholinergic neurons in the nucleus basalis. Ann Neurol 1981; 10(2): 122–6.

18. Jann MW. Rivastigmine, a new-generation cholinesterase inhibitor for the treatment of Alzheimer's disease. Pharmacotherapy 2000; 20(01): 1–12.

19. Muramoto O, Sugishita M, Sugita H et al. Effect of physostigmine on constructional and memory tasks in Alzheimer's disease. Arch Neurol 1979; 36(8): 501–3.

20. Davis KL, Thal LJ, Gamzu ER, et al. A double-blind, placebo-controlled multicenter study of tacrine for Alzheimer's disease. The Tacrine Collaborative Study Group. N Engl J Med 1992; 327(18): 1253–9.

21. Stahl SM. The new cholinesterase inhibitors for Alzheimer's disease, Part 1: their similarities are different. J Clin Psychiatry 2000; 61(10): 710–11.

22. Stahl SM. The new cholinesterase inhibitors for Alzheimer's disease, Part 2: illustrating their mechanisms of action. J Clin Psychiatry 2000; 61(11): 813–14.

23. Winblad B, Grossberg G, Frolich L et al. IDEAL: a 6-month, double-blind, placebo-controlled study of the first skin patch for Alzheimer disease. Neurology 2007; 69(Suppl 1):S14–S22.

24. Farlow MR. NMDA receptor antagonists. A new therapeutic approach for Alzheimer's disease. Geriatrics 2004; 59(6): 22–7.

25. Rogers SL, Farlow MR, Doody RS et al. A 24-week, double-blind, placebo-controlled trial of donepezil in patients with Alzheimer's disease. Neurology 1998; 50(1): 136–45.

26. Rosler M, Anand R, Cicin-Sain A et al. Efficacy and safety of rivastigmine in patients with Alzheimer's disease:

international randomised controlled trial. BMJ 1999; 318(7184): 633–8.

27. Wilcock GK, Lilienfeld S, Gaens E, on behalf of the Galantamine International-1 Study Group. Efficacy and safety of galantamine in patients with mild to moderate Alzheimer's disease: a multicentre randomised controlled trial. BMJ 2000; 321: 1–7.

28. Winblad B, Engedal K, Soininen H et al. A 1-year, randomized, placebo-controlled study of donepezil in patients with mild to moderate AD. Neurology 2001; 57(3): 489–95.

29. Raskind MA, Peskind ER, Wessel T et al. Galantamine USA-1 Study Group. Galantamine in AD: A 6-month randomized placebo-controlled trial with a 6-month extension. Neurology 2000; 54(12): 2261–8.

30. Doody RS, Geldmacher DS, Gordon B et al. Open-label, multicenter, phase 3 extension study of the safety and efficacy of donepezil in patients with Alzheimer disease. Arch Neurol 2001; 58(3): 427–33.

31. Rogers SL, Doody RS, Pratt RD et al. Long-term efficacy and safety of donepezil in the treatment of Alzheimer's disease: final analysis of a US multicentre open-label study. Eur Neuropsychopharmacol 2000; 10(3): 195–203.

32. Emre M. Switching cholinesterase inhibitors in patients with Alzheimer's disease. Int J Clin Pract Suppl 2002; 127: 64–72.

33. Mayor S. NICE recommends drugs for moderate Alzheimer's disease. BMJ 2006; 332(7535): 195.

34. Baudry M, Lynch G. Remembrance of arguments past: how well is the glutamate receptor hypothesis of LTP holding up after 20 years? Neurobiol Learn Mem 2001; 76: 284–97.

35. Meldrum BS, Garthwaite J. Excitatory amino acid neurotoxicity and neurodegenerative disease. Trends Pharmacol Sci 1990; 11: 993–6.

36. Reisberg B, Doody R, Stoffler A et al. Memantine in moderate to severe Alzheimer's disease. N Engl J Med 2003; 348: 1333–41.

37. Forest Laboratories I. A randomized, double-blind, placebo-controlled evaluation of the safety and efficacy of memantine in patients with moderate to severe dementia of the Alzheimer's type. 2005. http://www.forestclinicaltrials.com/CTR/CTRController/CTRCompletedListStudies

38. Tariot PN, Farlow MR, Grossberg GT et al. Memantine treatment in patients with moderate to severe Alzheimer disease already receiving donepezil: a randomized controlled trial. JAMA 2004; 291(3): 317–24.

39. Spector A, Orrell M, Davies S et al. Reality orientation for dementia. Cochrane Database Syst Rev. 2000; (4): CD001119.

40. Vink AC, Birks JS, Bruinsma MS et al. Music therapy for people with dementia. Cochrane Database Syst Rev 2004; (3): CD003477.

41. Holtzer R, Scarmeas N, Wegesin DJ et al. Depressive symptoms in Alzheimer's disease: natural course and temporal relation to function and cognitive status. J Am Geriatr Soc 2005; (12): 2083–9.

42. Petrovic M, De Paepe P, Van Bortel L. Pharmacotherapy of depression in old age. Acta Clin Belg 2005; 60(3): 150–6.

43. Boustani M, Watson L. The interface of depression and dementia. Psychiatric Times 2004, XXI: issue 3.

44. http://www.fda.gov/cder/drug/infopage/antipsychotics. Site visited in June 2006.

45. Olin JT, Fox LS, Pawluczyk S et al. A pilot randomized trial of carbamazepine for behavioral symptoms in treatment-resistant outpatients with Alzheimer disease. Am J Geriatr Psychiatry 2001; 9(4): 400–5.

46. Scarpini E, Scheltens P, Feldman H. Treatment of Alzheimer's disease: current status and new perspectives. Lancet Neurol 2003; 2: 1539–47.

47. Siemers ER, Quinn JF, Kaye J et al. Effects of a gamma-secretase inhibitor in a randomized study of patients with Alzheimer disease. Neurology 2006; 66(4): 602–4.

48. Schenk D, Barbour R, Dunn W et al. Immunization with amyloid-beta attenuates Alzheimer-disease-like pathology in the PDAPP mouse. Nature 1999; 400(6740): 173–7.

49. Orgogozo JM, Gilman S, Dartigues JF et al. Subacute meningoencephalitis in a subset of patients with AD after Abeta42 immunization. Neurology 2003; 61(1): 46–54.

50. Gilman S, Koller M, Black RS et al. Clinical effects of Abeta immunization (AN1792) in patients with AD in an interrupted trial. Neurology 2005; 64(9): 1553–62.

51. Nicoll JA, Wilkinson D, Holmes C et al. Neuropathology of human Alzheimer disease after immunization with amyloid-beta peptide: a case report. Nat Med 2003; 9(4): 448–52.

52. Du Y, Dodel R, Hampel H et al. Reduced levels of amyloid beta-peptide antibody in Alzheimer disease. Neurology 2000; 57: 801–5.

53. Dodel R, Hampel H, Depboylu C et al. Human antibodies against amyloid beta peptide: a potential treatment for Alzheimer's disease. Ann Neurol 2002; 52: 253–6.

54. Dodel RC, Du Y, Depboylu C et al. Intravenous immunoglobulins containing antibodies against beta-amyloid for the treatment of Alzheimer's disease. J Neurol Neurosurg Psychiatry 2004; 75: 1472–4.

55. Soto C. Protein misfolding and disease; protein refolding and therapy. FEBS Lett 2001; 498(2–3): 204–7.

56. McLaurin J, Kierstead ME, Brown ME et al. Cyclohexanehexol inhibitors of Abeta aggregation prevent and reverse Alzheimer phenotype in a mouse model. Nat Med 2006; 12(7): 80–8.

57. Gervais F. GAG mimetics: potential to modify underlying disease process in AD. Neurobiol Aging 2004; 25: S11–12.

58. Aisen PS, Mehran M, Poole R et al. Clinical data on Alzhemed after 12 months of treatment in patients with mild to moderate Alzheimer's disease [abstract]. Neurobiol Aging 2004; 25: 20.

59. Cherny RA, Atwood CS, Xilinas ME et al. Treatment with a copper-zinc chelator markedly and rapidly inhibits beta-amyloid accumulation in Alzheimer's disease transgenic mice. Neuron 2001; 30: 665–76.

60. Ritchie CW, Bush AI, Mackinnon A, et al. Metal-protein attenuation with iodochlor-hydroxyquin (clioquinol) targeting Abeta mechanisms, amyloid deposition and toxicity in Alzheimer disease: a pilot phase 2 clinical trial. Arch Neurol 2003; 60: 1685–91.

61. Sano M, Ernesto C, Thomas RG et al. A controlled trial of selegiline, alpha-tocopherol, or both as treatment for Alzheimer's disease. The Alzheimer's Disease Cooperative Study. N Engl J Med 1997; 336(17): 1216–22.

62. Petersen RC, Thomas RG, Grundman M et al. Vitamin E and donepezil for the treatment of mild cognitive impairment. N Engl J Med 2005; 352(23): 2379–88.

63. Miller ER 3rd, Pastor-Barriuso R, Dalal D et al. Meta-analysis: high-dosage vitamin E supplementation may increase all-cause mortality. Ann Intern Med 2005; 142(1): 37–46.

64. Loeb MB, Molloy DW, Smieja M et al. A randomized, controlled trial of doxycycline and rifampin for patients with Alzheimer's disease. J Am Geriatr Soc 2004; 52(3): 381–7.

65. Aisen PS. The potential of anti-inflammatory drugs for the treatment of Alzheimer's disease. Lancet Neurol 2002; 1: 279–84.

66. Shobab LA, Hsiung G-YR, Feldman HH. Cholesterol in Alzheimer's disease. Lancet Neurol 2005; 4: 841–52.

67. Sparks DL, Sabbagh MN, Connor DJ et al. Atorvastatin for the treatment of mild to moderate Alzheimer disease: preliminary results. Arch Neurol 2005; 62: 753–7.

68. Satou T, Itoh T, Tamai Y et al. Neurotrophic effects of FPF-1070 (Cerebrolysin®) on cultured neurons from chicken embryo dorsal root ganglia, ciliary ganglia, and sympathetic trunks. J Neural Transm 2000; 107: 1253–62.

69. Akai F, Hiruma S, Sato T. Neurotrophic factor-like effect of FPF1070 on septal cholinergic neurons after transection of fimbria-fornix in the rat brain. Histol Histopathol 1992; 7: 213–21.

70. Rockenstein E, Torrance M, Mante M et al. Cerebrolysin decreases amyloid-b production by regulating amyloid protein precursor maturation in a transgenic model of Alzheimer's disease. J Neurosci Res 2006; 83: 1252–61.

71. Ruether E, Humann R, Kinzler E et al. A 28-week, double-blind, placebo-controlled study with Cerebrolysin in patients with mild to moderate Alzheimer's disease. Int Clin Psychopharmacol 2001; 16: 253–63.

72. Panisset M, Gauthier S, Moessler H et al. Cerebrolysin in Alzheimer's disease: a randomized, double-blind, placebo-controlled trial with a neurotrophic agent. J Neural Transm 2002; 109: 1089–104.

73. Muresanu DF, Rainer M, Moessler H. Imporved global function and activities of daily living in patients with AD: a placebo-controlled clinical study with the neurotrophic agent Cerebrolysin. J Neural Transm 2002; 62(Suppl): 277–85.

74. Alvarez XA, Cacabelos R, Laredo M et al. A 24-week, double-blind, placebo-controlled study of three dosages of Cerebrolysin in patients with mild to moderate Alzheimer's disease. Euro J Neurol 2006; 13: 43–54.

CHAPTER 8

Alzheimer's disease: the future
Joyce Lin H Yeo and Howard H Feldman

INTRODUCTION

With the projected increase in the prevalence of Alzheimer's disease (AD) as Western society ages, the sense of urgency arising from diagnosis and treatment needs is becoming greater than ever. There will be myriad considerations related to the unprecedented number of Alzheimer sufferers in the future. From the social perspective, there will be housing and care needs which carry significant financial implications. The increased burden of care will alter family networks and societal structure as a whole. Medical issues arising from dementia such as vulnerability to delirium, malnutrition, pressure sores, and hospitalizations will place an enormous strain on healthcare resources. Clearly the key to managing will be through advances in research and implementation of strategies to cope with rising demands in health and social needs. As has been emphasized in this Atlas, there has been more progress in the elucidation of the cause and treatment of this illness in the past 15 years than in the previous century. This augurs well for a continued accelerated pace of research, however research progress will still require the important step of translation to clinical practice. Having the first approved symptomatic treatments for AD allows optimism that further therapeutic progress will follow. Advances in neuroimaging have provided new insights into the pathologic changes which occur in AD and biomarkers are being developed for early diagnosis and monitoring disease progression. Here we summarize a few key areas which hold promise for the future and discuss the broader implications of an aging society with increased numbers of patients with AD.

GENOMICS AND PROTEOMICS

The elucidation of genetic defects in familial autosomal dominant AD has been integral to research progress in the last two decades. Mutations on chromosome 21, 14 and 1 (APP, PSN1 and PSN2)[1,2] have led the way. From these discoveries it has been possible to develop transgenic animal models, knowledge of which has allowed new insights into the pathogenic disease mechanisms and the development of new therapies. It is not clear how many future candidate genes with autosomal dominant or other inheritance pathways remain to be discovered in AD.

Sporadic AD is heterogeneous. Apart from the identification of apolipoprotein E (APOE), the search for other deterministic genes has not been as fruitful as expected.[3,4] Currently it is estimated that half of the genetic profile for sporadic AD has been accounted for, allowing that further genetic breakthroughs can be anticipated. Further work is being carried out examining single nucleotide polymorphisms (single base differences within the genome, e.g. APOE) which are likely to provide useful tools for further dissection of the genetic risk factors of AD. Genome wide linkage or linkage disequilibrium studies have also provided data for the existence of other promising candidate genes, e.g. insulin-degrading enzyme gene on chromosome 10 and various gene polymorphisms on chromosome 12 (see Figure 8.1).[1,5,6]

As these efforts intensify and the need for large-scale gene variation analysis increases, gene chip arrays have developed to become a means of analyzing hundreds of genomes on a single chip at one time.[7,8]

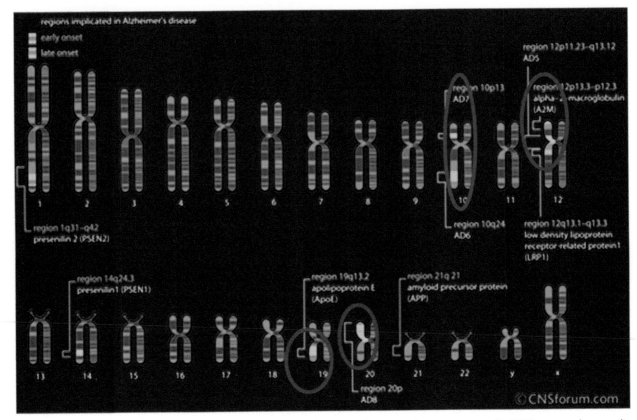

Figure 8.1   The majority of these familial cases are due to mutations in the amyloid precursor protein (APP) gene and presenilin (PSEN) 1 and 2, two genes encoding 7 transmembrane domain proteins. The remaining cases present at a later age and display more complex inheritance. Susceptibility loci (AD5–8) have been mapped to chromosomes 10, 12, and 20. Candidate genes have been identified within AD6 and AD8. The gene for insulin-degrading enzyme, a metallopeptidase that can degrade a number of peptides including β-amyloid, is located within AD6 and the CST3 gene, encoding cystatin C, an inhibitor of cysteine proteases that has been shown to co-deposit with APP in AD brains, maps within AD8. Associations have been demonstrated with the apoEε4 allele on chromosome 19 and a polymorphism in A2M and LRP1. Reproduced with permission from www.cnsforum.com.

Parallel to the study of genes is the study of the products of gene expression and their post-translational modifications. This study of proteins or proteomics has grown out of the elucidation of genomic expression and is making inroads into AD biomarker development as well as new therapeutic targets. New proteomic technologies allow the ability to analyze thousands of proteins in a single sample, increasing specificity and reproducibility.[9]

Applications of proteomics in AD are in their very early phases, but given that AD is a complex disease, it is possible that a whole pattern reflecting disease state, akin to a 'fingerprint', is more accurate than the presence of any single biomarker. The way forward would then be to retrace the genomic determinants of the abnormal protein expression and consider pharmacogenomic therapy at an early stage before neuropathologic changes occur.

BIOMARKERS

An integral step in the future will need to be directed at developing more reliable and practical biomarkers with clinical utility. According to the Reagan Working Group Consensus of 2003, biomarkers should be inexpensive, non-invasive, reproducible, and simple to perform.[10] Previous and current endeavors have concentrated on cerebrospinal fluid and neuroimaging techniques as a closer reflection of the pathologic process in AD brain. The ideal biomarker should act as a window to disease and permit a way of visualizing illness directly.

CSF tau and β-amyloid

CSF markers for tracking the pathologic processes of AD have been reported in numerous research studies over the last decade. Three of the most promising biomarkers in CSF (P-tau, T-tau and β-amyloid) have high sensitivity for differentiating early AD from normal aging, depression, alcoholic dementia, and Parkinson's disease, but lower specificity against other dementias such as frontotemporal degeneration and Lewy body dementia.[11,12] Combining a battery of CSF biomarkers may improve diagnostic accuracy, for example combining CSF β-amyloid and total tau has been reported to increase specificity to 85%.[13]

Despite these promising results, the clinical utility of CSF tau and β-amyloid remains uncertain. There is significant overlap between AD and non-AD individuals, and measurement methods differ across studies. These methodologic inconsistencies limit the diagnostic usefulness of these biomarkers presently. Clearly there is a need for increased research collaboration and standardizing methodologies. Further prospective studies of CSF tau and β-amyloid are also needed to decipher the role of each and to determine the potential diagnostic utility of these measurements.

Other biomarkers

Analyses of blood, serum, and urine have also been investigated, however these provide only an indirect view of brain function. Isoprostanes and sulfatides are markers of oxidative stress and lipid composition thought to be indicative of AD pathogenesis. Their development as putative biomarkers is currently viewed as promising. However, inconsistencies exist due to assay variability and selection criteria,[14,15] and there is currently inadequate evidence supporting their use.[16,17]

NEUROIMAGING

Over the past two decades, advances in neuroimaging have provided the greatest insights into brain structure and function in AD. The initial breakthrough with CT has now been surpassed by MRI and PET. The National Institute of Health has funded the Alzheimer's Disease Neuroimaging Initiative (ADNI) to set standards for image acquisition, the development of a data repository, and the analysis of best imaging approaches for clinical trials.[18]

With MRI neuroimaging it has become possible to measure both whole brain and hippocampal volumes as well as their rates of atrophy. These techniques have been able to distinguish normal from AD but are still finding their place in differential dementia diagnosis. Evolving MR techniques which determine the motional properties of brain water in living tissue such as diffusion weighted imaging and diffusion tensor imaging may permit greater resolution and differentiation of AD from vascular and other related dementias. Hippocampal and entorhinal cortex measurements have been shown to predict progression to AD in asymptomatic individuals and those with mild cognitive impairment allowing that foreseeably the application of longitudinal structural magnetic resonance imaging (MRI) will be used as a surrogate marker of disease progression (see Figure 8.2). This should facilitate the evaluation of new therapies. Further application of this technology in longitudinal studies in subjects with few or no symptoms is also beginning to yield promising results, enhancing the predictive utility of this modality.[19–21]

Functional MR provides a powerful tool to investigate brain activation patterns in response to cognitive processing. It has the advantages of high temporal and spatial resolution and may be applicable in the development of cognitive stress tests that may identify individuals at risk of AD (see Figure 8.3). Recent studies have demonstrated its potential in MCI patients and in individuals carrying the apoE4 allele.[23,24]

For these advancing techniques to reach clinical practise, there will need to be robust and more accessible automated methods for quantitative assessment of images. Currently the imaging data files are very large and require sophisticated multidisciplinary analyses out of reach in most clinical settings.

Positron emission tomography (PET) has also provided unique insights into patterns of impairment that occur at the earliest stages of disease and together with the use of novel molecular probes, is revealing the location of AD pathology *in vivo*. PET with the metabolic tracer [18F]fluorodeoxyglucose or FDG measures the brain metabolism of glucose which is generally coupled with cerebral blood flow. It has reasonable to good discriminatory ability to distinguish between AD from controls with a disease pattern of bitemporal and biparietal hypometabolism and hypoperfusion in AD patients as demonstrated in Figure 8.4.

An exciting new era has opened with the development of radioligands that can be safely administered to humans and can tag aggregating proteins including

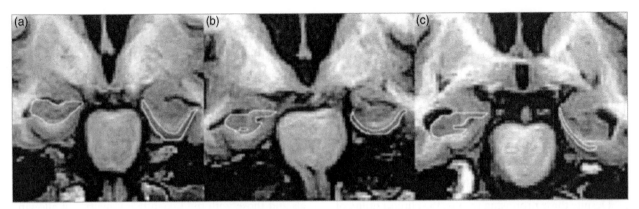

Figure 8.2 Entorhinal cortex (ERC) (right) and hippocampal (left) volume measurement in volumetric magnetization prepared rapid acquisition gradient echo (MP-RAGE) images. (a) Normal cognition (NC); (b) mild cognitive impairment (MCI); (c) Alzheimer's disease (AD). Reproduced from[22] with permission from Elsevier.

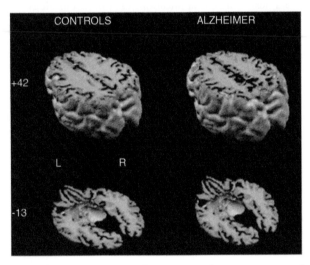

Figure 8.3 Relative contribution maps from group general linear model (GLM) analysis in 14 AD patients (right side) and 14 age-matched healthy control subjects (left side). Red color indicates task-related activation in favor of a visuospatial task (discrimination of angle sizes) vs a visuomotor control task. Both groups did not differ in their performance on the tasks. AD patients revealed less task-related activation in the bilateral superior parietal cortex (upper part of the picture) and more activation in the left inferior temporal cortex when compared with the control group (lower part of the picture). Reproduced from [25] with permission from BMJ publishing group.

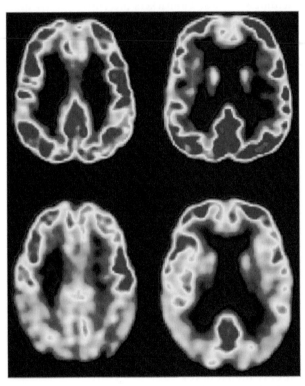

Figure 8.4 FDG-PET data from an older control subject (top) and a patient with probable Alzheimer's disease (bottom), illustrating prominent temporo-parietal hypometabolism. Reproduced with permission from [20]. Copyright © 2005, American Society for Experimental NeuroTherapeutics. All rights reserved.

β-amyloid and tau. There are two compound tracers: Pittsburgh compound-B (carbon-11-labelled PIB), which labels β-amyloid (as illustrated in Figure 8.5), and [18F]FDDNP (fluorine-18-labelled FDDNP), which labels both β-amyloid and tau. Both have been used in humans and have demonstrated the characteristic retention in AD subjects that is consistent with AD pathology.[26,27]

Forseeably, there will be other additional compounds to be developed for PET.[28] The potential of these compounds lies in their ability to quantify AD pathology *in vivo* for the first time. The combination of these compounds with other biochemical and genetic biomarkers is a powerful addition to the current battery

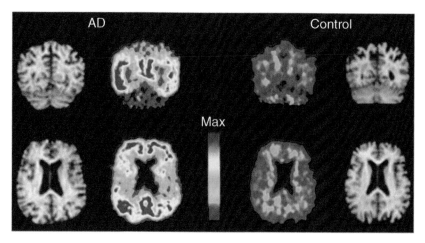

Figure 8.5 *In vivo* PET-based detection of β-amyloid. Increased retention of Pittsburgh compound-B (PIB) is found in frontal and temporo-parietal regions in patients with clinical AD. Reproduced with permission from [20]. Copyright © 2006, American Society for Experimental NeuroTherapeutics. All rights reserved.

of biomarkers. An early report using PIB with PET in conjunction with CSF amyloid beta 1–42 has been documented demonstrating that greater amounts of β-amyloid-containing plaques in the brain were associated with lower levels of amyloid beta 1–42 in CSF.[29] Many methodologic issues remain unresolved and the clinical value of these tracers has yet to be realized, but their potential as a surrogate marker for AD is promising.

Single photon emission computer tomography (SPECT) with Tc-99m ligands demonstrates temporo-parietal hypoperfusion in AD patients, although it is less sensitive and specific than PET. Ligands which trace β-amyloid and tau are also being developed for SPECT although this has been limited to *in vitro* studies so far.[30]

THERAPY

The last decade has witnessed the first successful development in therapeutics for AD. This success has concentrated within symptomatic treatments based on neurochemical targets. The door is opening to treatments linked more definitively to disease pathogenesis and several are under development at various stages and with a variety of treatment goals in mind (see Figure 8.6).

Overall the focus of treatment with a disease-modifying intent will be increasingly moving towards early and incipient AD with a view of preventing or attenuating disease before symptoms occur.

Symptomatic treatment

The most widely employed current strategy for symptomatic treatment of AD is the replacement and modulation of neurotransmitters (illustrated in Figure 8.7). The

acetylcholinesterase inhibitors (AchEIs) and the NMDA uncompetitive antagonist memantine have been approved for the symptoms of AD. They provide modest but clinically meaningful symptomatic benefits in cognition, ADL, and behavior.

Disease-modifying treatment

The development of therapies which target the pathologic processes in AD are evolving to include immunotherapies, amyloid-lowering approaches, and tau-based treatments as well as antioxidant and anti-apoptotic approaches.

Targeting β-amyloid formation, deposition, and clearance (see Figure 8.8)

(1) γ- and β-secretase inhibitors

The γ- and β- secretases are proteases which cleave amyloid precursor protein, producing β-amyloid. Inhibitors of these enzymes are being developed, notably γ-secretase inhibitors (R-Flurbiprofen and LY450139 dihydrate), which have proceeded from phase 1 to phase 2 trials.[33,34]

There have been studies of β-secretase in animals proving that inhibition of the enzyme can be achieved without toxicity,[35,36] however the selectivity of inhibition, stability, and ease of blood–brain barrier penetration and cellular uptake are issues which remain to be addressed for β-secretase inhibitors.

(2) Amyloid antiaggregant therapies and β-sheet breakers

A seminal pathologic event in Alzheimer's disease is the misfolding and aggregation of normal amyloid beta

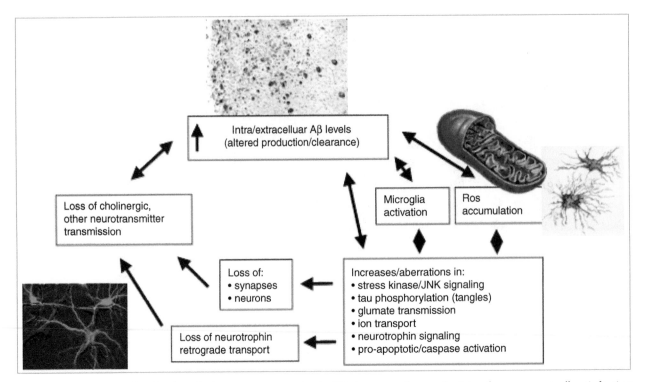

Figure 8.6   Overview of pathophysiologic processes occurring in AD. A perspective emphasizing the many mutually reinforcing pathologic processes in AD suggests that neuroprotective strategies, inhibiting as many of these processes as possible, will likely be required. From [31] copyright © 2004, American Society for Experimental NeuroTherapeutics. All rights reserved.

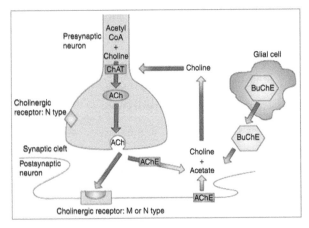

Figure 8.7   Functional features of the cholinergic system. Ach = acetylcholine; AChE = acetylcholinesterase; BuChE = butyrylcholinesterase; ChAT = choline acetyltransferase; CoA = coenzyme A. Reprinted from [32] with permission from Elsevier.

peptide into β-sheet-rich oligomers that are neurotoxic and deposit as insoluble senile neuritic plaques in AD brains. Newly engineered synthetic β-sheet breaker peptides bind soluble amyloid and prevent or reverse this abnormal conformational change. Application of these peptides in transgenic mice has

been shown to demonstrate a reduction of β-amyloid in mouse brain.[37]

Drugs currently under testing which also target this process include tramiprosate (Alzhemed™), which works by interfering with glycosaminoglycans associated with the binding and aggregation of β-amyloid. It is currently in phase 3 trials.[38]

Clioquinol, a retired hydrophobic antibiotic with brain penetrating and Cu/Zn chelating properties, is another potential agent that works by inhibiting copper and zinc ions from binding to β-amyloid, thus preventing its accumulation. It is currently in phase 2 trials. Its safety however, must still be established.[39]

(3) Statins

Excess brain cholesterol has been associated with increased formation and deposition of amyloid beta peptide from amyloid precursor protein in AD. The HMG-CoA reductase inhibitors (statins) have been considered therapeutically as they may both lower cholesterol and have a role in APP processing.[40,41] A number of trials are in progress and more are needed before definite conclusions can be drawn. A pilot study

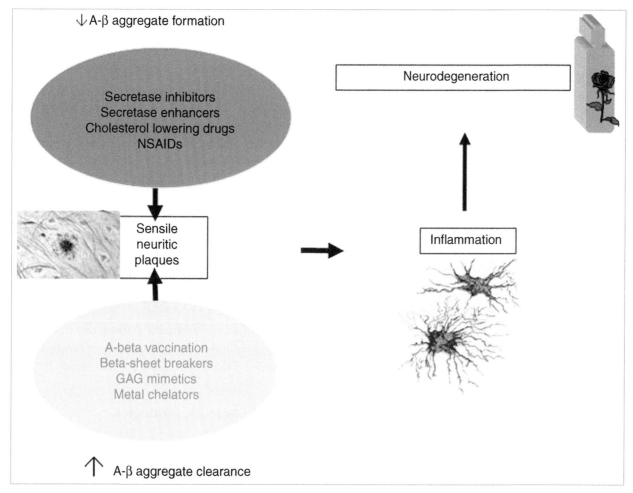

Figure 8.8 This figure summarizes the main hypothesized pathological processes and the related therapeutic approaches to AD. Modified from [32] copyright ©2003, with permission from Elsevier.

of atorvastatin looked encouraging and has spurred large-scale trials that are in progress.[42]

(4) Immunotherapies and vaccines

Over the last 5 years there has been significant progress in developing immunotherapeutic approaches to AD. The underlying rationale is that the host immune system can be activated to specific targets. This led to the development of amyloid beta vaccines which have been successful in transgenic mice overproducing amyloid beta (TGCRND8) (illustrated in Figures 8.9, 8.10 and 8.11).

In this TGCRND8 mouse model amyloid beta was both cleared and its deposition prevented. Unfortunately, the first human trial came to a halt in 2002 when an autoimmune encephalitis was identified in 6% of subjects.[45] Nevertheless, the neuropathologic reports have suggested that a substantive reduction of amyloid beta deposition was achieved with this vaccine.[46] Despite this initial setback immunotherapy seems promising for the future. In an effort to bypass earlier

problems, researchers are experimenting with passive immunization and novel Aβ peptide immunogens.[47]

Targeting cell signaling pathways and tangle formation

(1) Stress kinase signaling inhibitors

The stimulation of stress-activated kinases, especially the c Jun N-terminal kinase (JNK), has been recognized as an early event in neuronal degeneration associated with AD. Evidence *in vitro* that inhibition of JNK activation inhibits amyloid beta deposition has led to the development of compounds that block stress kinase signaling. CEP 1347 is currently being investigated in clinical trials for Parkinson's and is likely to be a candidate agent for AD trials.[31]

(2) Tau phosphorylation inhibitors

The hyperphosphorylation of tau leads to unstable microtubules and neuronal dysfunction. There is evidence that glycogen synthase kinase 3-β (GSK-β)

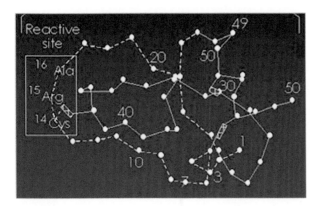

Figure 8.9 Structure of the amyloid beta peptide used as a vaccine in initial studies. Reproduced with kind permission from [43] and [44].

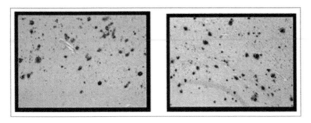

Figure 8.10 On the left is accumulation of amyloid deposits in human brain with AD at 70 years of age. On the right is accumulation of amyloid deposits in transgenic mouse (TgCRND8) at equivalent age (70 to 100 days). (Reproduced with kind permission from [43] and [44].

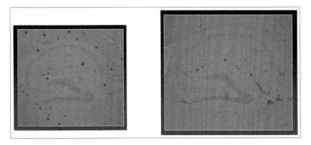

Figure 8.11 Immunization with the amyloid beta peptide reduces tissue change in Alzheimer's mouse model: before and after (image on the right). Reproduced with kind permission from St George Hyslop (McLaurin et al. Nature Genetics 2002; 8(11): 1263–9[44]; Janus et al. Nature 2000; 408(6815): 979–82[43]).

phosphorylates tau and is upregulated in AD, resulting in a therapeutic interest in GSK inhibitors. Valproate and lithium, both of which inhibit GSK, have been postulated as treatments that might improve and modify AD.[31] Phosphatase 2A, mitogen activated kinase/extracellular reactive kinase1/2 (MAPK/ERK1/2) and cyclin

dependent kinase 5 (CdK5) have also been implicated in the hyperphosphorylation of tau and have been proposed as potential therapeutic targets.

(3) Caspase inhibitors

Programmed cell death, or apoptosis, is executed by a series of cysteine aspartyl proteases (caspases) that form a proteolytic cascade. Each caspase functions either to activate downstream caspases by proteolytic cleavage and/or to proteolytically cleave cellular substrates. Increased levels of apoptosis and caspase activity are frequently observed at sites of cellular damage in both acute (e.g. myocardial infarction, stroke, sepsis) and chronic diseases (e.g. AD, Parkinson's, and Huntington's disease). In turn, inhibition of caspase activity to reduce cell death and tissue damage may be therapeutically beneficial in AD.

Many of these compounds demonstrate efficacy in a wide range of animal models; however, it remains to be determined if this will be applicable in humans.[48]

Other therapeutic strategies

Antioxidant therapies

Oxidative stress causes damage to cell function with aging and in cellular studies appears to precede the pathologic hallmarks in AD brain. As a result, various antioxidants have been examined, notably vitamin E, coenzyme Q10, and curcumin. Cross-sectional longitudinal studies exploring the relationship between vitamin E and AD risk have not identified a consistent benefit and a recent meta-analysis has suggested that there may be an increased mortality associated with vitamin E use. Preliminary studies suggest that coenzyme Q10 and curcumin may delay AD due to their antioxidant properties and both are undergoing phase 1 and phase 2 trials, respectively.[49–51]

Anti-inflammatory drugs

Retrospective epidemiologic studies have consistently reported a reduction in risk of AD associated with the chronic use of non-steroidal anti-inflammatory drugs (NSAIDS).[52] In turn, there have been a large number of placebo controlled, randomized trials to investigate the efficacy of various anti-inflammatory approaches including NSAIDs. Most of the studies have not demonstrated efficacy in AD treatment, though their potential utility has not been fully evaluated.[53–55]

Other anti-inflammatory approaches have focused on the modulation of astrocytes involved in the inflammatory process and the inhibition of glial activation. ONO-2506, a neuroprotective agent which modulates astrocyte activity, is currently undergoing phase III trials. Aminopyridazines which inhibit inflammatory cytokine pathways as well as glial activation has been found to reduce amyloid load in transgenic mice.

Neurotrophins

Given the degenerative nature of AD there has been interest in supplementing neurotrophic factors in AD. It has been postulated that synaptic failure occurs early in AD and neurotrophins could potentially assist in synapse stabilization and function.[31]

A phase 1 clinical trial utilized a unique *ex vivo* gene therapy approach to deliver nerve growth factor directly to the basal forebrain of AD patients. Despite the need for further testing, their report illustrated a mild but significant therapeutic benefit of NGF for the treatment of AD and provided important data concerning the safety and efficacy of *ex vivo* gene therapy in humans (see Figure 8.12).

Hormonal treatment

The relationship between hormones and Alzheimer's disease has been the focus of much research. This has concentrated mainly on estrogen due to observational studies that hormone replacement therapy may prevent the development of AD. Recent trials, however, failed to show any benefit in preventing or alleviating the disease although its potential has not been fully evaluated. Recently other hormones, notably luteinizing hormone, have been targeted as an important causative factor in the development of AD, leading to the development of a gonadotropin releasing hormone agonist designed to reduce the levels of luteinizing hormone currently undergoing phase 3 trials.[57]

FUTURE SOCIETAL AND ECONOMIC IMPLICATIONS OF AD

The increase in prevalence of AD brings with it huge societal and economic implications. In Canada, as an example, the cost of healthcare is predicted to escalate from 4 billion to over 12 billion dollars by the year 2031 (see Figure 8.13). The most significant contributing cost

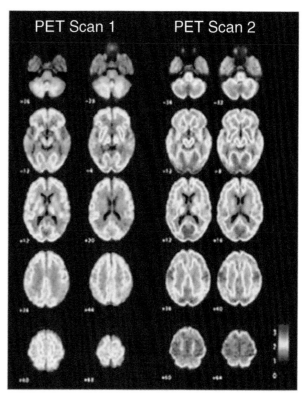

Figure 8.12 Averaged FDG-PET scan images in four subjects treated with NGF, overlaid on standardized MRI templates. Representative axial sections, with 6–8 months between first and second scan, showing widespread interval increases in brain metabolism. Flame scale indicates FDG use/100 g tissue/min; red color indicates more FDG use than blue. Image courtesy of University of California – San Diego. Reproduced with permission from Tuszynski et al. A phase 1 clinical trial of nerve growth factor gene therapy for Alzheimer disease. Nature Medicine 2005; 11(5): 551.[56]

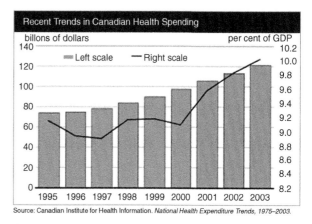

Figure 8.13 Increasing concerns are being raised as to whether these trends are sustainable, concerns that are made more acute by future pressures on the health system, including the aging of Canada's population. These trends are generalizable across Western society as a whole. Reproduced with permission from the Canadian Institute for Health Information, National Health Expenditure Trends 1975–2003.

will be the institutional care costs, while the need for assistance with everyday activities of daily living from professionals, family, and friends in the community setting will grow incrementally. Worryingly, these costs are reflected across most of the Western world. Global population aging trends in most of the rest of the world will result in shrinking workforces struggling to cope with looking after the elderly with dementia impacting on the economic growth and development in these countries.

Despite optimism on the research front, the reality is that it will take time for research knowledge to be incorporated into clinical practise, and to be integrated into policy, practise, program, and funding decisions. In the foreseeable future, the increasingly complex health needs seem destined to reach a crisis as healthcare systems are restructured and institutional residential beds are reduced. The expansion of community-based services could offset the losses of residential care. Whether this will be sufficient to manage intensive, long-term healthcare needs is uncertain. A number of studies have shown the advantages of substituting home care services for more costly institutional services (e.g., hospital, residential care facilities).[58,59] Despite the increase in these services, it did not really benefit those who needed it most, the elderly with dementia and complex health needs. For example, with current health reform in the West, there has been a reduction of acute care beds, a shortening of length of hospital stay, an increase in outpatient surgery, and only modest increases to home care budgets. Home care is being changed from a chronic care support system for seniors to a medical support system for intensive post-acute care for hospital (including outpatient) discharges. Clearly, an appropriate expansion will be needed to provide the range of services the elderly with dementia are likely to need.[60]

Future provision of care for AD sufferers will require a national response and integration at all levels. Better training of health professionals has to be given resource priority if it is to sustain the inevitable demand for care facilities able to cope with complex needs (see Figures 8.14 and 8.15).

CONCLUSION

This *Atlas of Alzheimer's Disease* ends on a mixed note of excitement and apprehension. The excitement stems

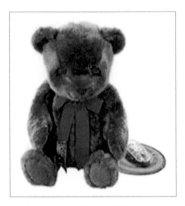

Figure 8.14 The future for Alzheimer's sufferers? This digital bear monitors patients' response times to spoken questions. It records how long they spend performing various tasks, before relaying conclusions to staff or alerting them to unexpected changes. The voice recognition interface helps remove the barriers presented by using traditional computers for similar tasks. The fur-covered robotic assistant, simply known as 'Teddy', hides a microcomputer and a local network connection. This bear features in a 106 bed facility run by Matsushita Electronics, which incorporates the latest in technology to help care for Japan's aging population. Reproduced with kind permission from Japan Inc Magazine, 2002.

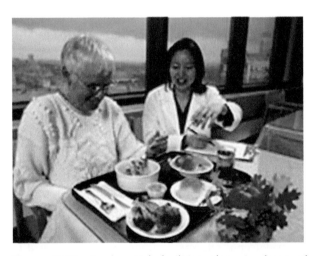

Figure 8.15 As hospital facilities close in favor of community-based care, adequate planning and resource delivery is crucial to ensure increasingly complex needs are catered for. Reproduced with kind permission from www.turbophoto.com.

from the pace of research progress in AD and the potential for new and more definitive therapies. The apprehension grows from the aging world population with AD and the needs that this will create in all dimensions at a societal level. An integrated international effort must occur to ensure a better future for AD patients as we await research progress to provide new treatment opportunities to both prevent and treat AD.

REFERENCES

1. Serretti A, Artioli P, Quartesan R, De RD. Genes involved in Alzheimer's disease, a survey of possible candidates. J Alzheimers Dis 2005a; 7(4): 331–53.

2. St George-Hyslop PH, Petit A. Molecular biology and genetics of Alzheimer's disease. C R Biol 2005; 328(2), 119–30.

3. Breitner JC. APOE genotyping and Alzheimer's disease. Lancet 1996; 347(9009): 1184–85.

4. Blacker D, Haines JL, Rodes L et al. ApoE-4 and age at onset of Alzheimer's disease: the NIMH genetics initiative. Neurology 1997; 48(1): 139–47.

5. Poduslo SE, Yin X. Chromosome 12 and late-onset Alzheimer's disease. Neurosci Lett 2001; 310(2-3): 188–90.

6. Qiu WQ, Folstein MF. Insulin, insulin-degrading enzyme and amyloid-beta peptide in Alzheimer's disease: review and hypothesis. Neurobiol Aging 2006; 27(2): 190–8.

7. Pasinetti GM, Ho L. From cDNA microarrays to high-throughput proteomics. Implications in the search for preventive initiatives to slow the clinical progression of Alzheimer's disease dementia. Restor Neurol Neurosci 2001; 18(2-3): 137–42.

8. Marcotte ER, Srivastava LK, Quirion R. cDNA microarray and proteomic approaches in the study of brain diseases: focus on schizophrenia and Alzheimer's disease. Pharmacol Ther 2003; 100(1): 63–74.

9. Butterfield DA, Boyd-Kimball D. Proteomics analysis in Alzheimer's disease: new insights into mechanisms of neurodegeneration. Int Rev Neurobiol 2004; 61: 159–88.

10. Frank RA, Galasko D, Hampel H et al. Biological markers for therapeutic trials in Alzheimer's disease. Proceedings of the biological markers working group; NIA initiative on neuroimaging in Alzheimer's disease. Neurobiol Aging 2003; 24(4): 521–36.

11. Ganzer S, Arlt S, Schoder V et al. CSF-tau, CSF-Abeta1-42, ApoE-genotype and clinical parameters in the diagnosis of Alzheimer's disease: combination of CSF-tau and MMSE yields highest sensitivity and specificity. J Neural Transm 2003; 110(10): 1149–60.

12. Andreasen N, Blennow K. CSF biomarkers for mild cognitive impairment and early Alzheimer's disease. Clin Neurol Neurosurg 2005; 107(3): 165–173.

13. Ganzer S, Arlt S, Schoder V et al. CSF-tau, CSF-Abeta1-42, ApoE-genotype and clinical parameters in the diagnosis of Alzheimer's disease: combination of CSF-tau and MMSE yields highest sensitivity and specificity. J Neural Transm 2003; 110(10): 1149–60.

14. Reich EE, Markesbery WR, Roberts LJ et al. Quantification of F-ring and D-/E-ring isoprostanes and neuroprostanes in Alzheimer's disease. Adv Exp Med Biol 2001; 500: 253–6.

15. Kim KM, Jung BH, Paeng KJ et al. Increased urinary F(2)-isoprostane levels in the patient with Alzheimer's disease. Brain Res Bull 2004; 64(1): 47–51.

16. Han X, Holtzman M, McKeel DW, Jr et al. Substantial sulfatide deficiency and ceramide elevation in very early Alzheimer's disease: potential role in disease pathogenesis. J Neurochem 2002; 82(4): 809–18.

17. Irizarry MC. A turn of the sulfatide in Alzheimer's disease 2003; Ann Neurol 54(1), 7–8.

18. Mueller SG, Weiner MW, Thal LJ et al. The Alzheimer's disease neuroimaging initiative. Neuroimaging Clin N Am 2005; 15(4), 869–77, xi–xii.

19. Mosconi L, De SS, Rusinek H, Convit A, de Leon MJ. Magnetic resonance and PET studies in the early diagnosis of Alzheimer's disease. Expert Rev Neurother 2004; 4(5): 831–849.

20. Dickerson BC, Sperling RA. Neuroimaging biomarkers for clinical trials of disease-modifying therapies in Alzheimer's disease. NeuroRx 2005; 2(2): 348–360.

21. Bittner D, Gron G, Schirrmeister H, Reske SN, Riepe MW. [18F]FDG-PET in patients with Alzheimer's disease: marker of disease spread. Dement Geriatr Cogn Disord 2005; 19(1): 24–30.

22. Du, Shuff N, Ameud D. Magnetic resonance imaging of the entorhinal cortex and hippocampus in mild cognitive impairment and Alzheimer's disease. J Neurol Neurosurg Psychiatry 2001; 71(4): 441–7.

23. Bookheimer SY, Strojwas MH, Cohen MS et al. Patterns of brain activation in people at risk for Alzheimer's disease. N Engl J Med 2000; 343(7): 450–456.

24. Dickerson BC, Salat DH, Bates JF et al. Medial temporal lobe function and structure in mild cognitive impairment. Ann Neurol 2004; 56(1): 27–35.

25. Prvulovic D, Hubl D, Sack AT. Functional imaging of visuospatial processing in Alzheimer's disease. NeuroImage 2002; 17: 1403–14.

26. Sair HI, Doraiswamy PM, Petrella JR. In vivo amyloid imaging in Alzheimer's disease. Neuroradiology 2004; 46(2): 93–104.

27. Okamura N, Suemoto T, Furumoto S et al. Quinoline and benzimidazole derivatives: candidate probes for in vivo imaging of tau pathology in Alzheimer's disease. J Neurosci 2005; 25(47): 10857–10862.

28. Verhoeff NP, Wilson AA, Takeshita S et al. In-vivo imaging of Alzheimer disease beta-amyloid with [11C]SB-13 PET. Am J Geriatr Psychiatry 2004; 12(6): 584–595.

29. Fagan AM, Mintun MA, Mach RH et al. Inverse relation between in vivo amyloid imaging load and cerebrospinal fluid Abeta(42) in humans. Ann Neurol 2006; 59(3): 512–9.

30. Kung MP, Hou C, Zhuang ZP et al. Binding of two potential imaging agents targeting amyloid plaques in postmortem brain tissues of patients with Alzheimer's disease. Brain Res 2004; 1025(1–2): 98–105.

31. Longo FM, Massa SM. Neuroprotective strategies in Alzheimer's disease. NeuroRx 2004; 1(1): 117–27.

32. Scarpini E, Scheltens, Feldman H. Treatment of Alzheimer's disease: current treatment and new perspectives. Lancet Neurol 2003; 2(9): 539–47.

33. Efficacy and safety of MPC-7869: a selective AB42-lowering agent in Alzheimer's disease (AD): Results of a 12-month Phase 2 trial and 1-year follow-on study. www.myriad.com accessed 23rd March 2006. Ref type: internet communication.

34. Siemers ER, Quinn J, Kaye J et al. Effects of a gamma-secretase inhibitor in a randomized study of patients with Alzheimer disease. Neurology 2006; 66(4): 602–4.

35. Vassar R. BACE1: the beta-secretase enzyme in Alzheimer's disease. J Mol Neurosci 2004; 23(1–2): 105–14.

36. Churcher I, Beher D. Gamma-secretase as a therapeutic target for the treatment of Alzheimer's disease. Curr Pharm Des 2005; 11(26): 3363–82.

37. Bieler S, Soto C. Beta-sheet breakers for Alzheimer's disease therapy. Curr Drug Targets 2004; 5(6): 553–8.

38. Tramiprosate (Alzhemed™) currently in large Phase III clinical trials in North America and Europe. www.neurochem.com, accessed 23rd March 2006. internet communication.

39. Regland B, Lehmann W, Abedini I et al. Treatment of Alzheimer's disease with clioquinol. Dement Geriatr Cogn Disord 2001; 12(6): 408–14.

40. Shobab LA, Hsiung GY, Feldman HH. Cholesterol in Alzheimer's disease. Lancet Neurol 2005; 4(12): 841–52.

41. Sjogren M, Mielke M, Gustafson D et al. Cholesterol and Alzheimer's disease – is there a relation? Mech Ageing Dev 2005;

42. Sparks DL, Sabbagh MN, Connor DJ et al. Atorvastatin for the treatment of mild to moderate Alzheimer disease: preliminary results. Arch Neurol 2005; 62(5): 753–7.

43. Janus C, Pearson J, McLawrin J et al. A beta peptide immunization reduces behavioural impairment and plaques in a model of Alzheimer's disease. Nature 2000; 408(6815): 979–82.

44. McLawrin JR, Cecal ME, Kierstead X et al. Therapeutically effective antibodies agtainst amyloid-β peptide target amyloid-β residues 4–10 and inhibit cytotoxicity and fibrilogenesis. Nature Genetics 2002; 8(11): 1263–9.

45. Orgogozo JM, Gilman S, Dartigues JF et al. Subacute meningoencephalitis in a subset of patients with AD after Abeta42 immunization. Neurology 2003; 61: 46–54.

46. Nicoll JA, Wilkinson D, Holmes C et al. Neuropathology of human Alzheimer disease after immunization with amyloid-beta peptide: a case report. Nature Med 2003; 9(4): 448–52.

47. Maier M, Seabrook TJ, Lazo ND et al. Short amyloid-beta (Abeta) immunogens reduce cerebral Abeta load and learning deficits in an Alzheimer's disease mouse model in the absence of an Abeta-specific cellular immune response. J Neurosci 2006; 26(18): 4717–28.

48. Cribbs DH, Poon WW, Rissman RA, Blurton-Jones M. Caspase-mediated degeneration in Alzheimer's disease. Am J Pathol 2004; 165(2): 353–5.

49. Beal MF. Mitochondrial dysfunction and oxidative damage in Alzheimer's and Parkinson's diseases and coenzyme Q10 as a potential treatment. J Bioenerg Biomembr 2004; 36(4): 381–6.

50. Ono K, Hasegawa K, Naiki H, Yamada M. Curcumin has potent anti-amyloidogenic effects for Alzheimer's beta-amyloid fibrils in vitro. J Neurosci Res 2004; 75(6): 742–50.

51. Ringman JM, Frautschy SA, Cole GM et al. A potential role of the curry spice curcumin in Alzheimer's disease. Curr Alzheimer Res 2005; 2(2): 131–6.

52. McGeer PL, Schulzer M, McGeer EG. Arthritis and anti-inflammatory agents as possible protective factors for Alzheimer's disease: a review of 17 epidemiologic studies. Neurology 1996; 47(2): 425–32.

53. Pasinetti GM. From epidemiology to therapeutic trials with antiinflammatory drugs in Alzheimer's disease: the role of NSAIDs and cyclooxygenase in beta-amyloidosis and clinical dementia. J Alzheimers Dis 2002; 4(5): 435–45.

54. Gasparini L, Ongini E, Wenk G. Non-steroidal anti-inflammatory drugs (NSAIDs) in Alzheimer's disease: old and new mechanisms of action. J Neurochem 2004; 91(3): 521–36.

55. Secko D. Can NSAIDs contribute to Alzheimer's disease? CMAJ 2005; 172(13): 1677.

56. Tuszynski MH, Thal L, Pay M et al. A phase 1 clinical trial of nerve growth factor gene therapy for Alzheimer disease. Nat Med 2005; 11(5): 551–5.

57. Casadesus G, Atwood CS, Zhu X et al. Evidence for the role of gonadotropin hormones in the development of Alzheimer disease. Cell Mol Life Sci 2005; 62(3): 293–8.

58. Chappell NL, Penning MJ. Sociology of aging in Canada: issues for the millennium. Can J Aging–Rev Can Vieillissement 2001; 20: 82–110.

59. McDowell I, Hill G, Lindsay J et al. Patterns and health effects of caring for people with dementia: the impact of changing cognitive and residential status. Gerontologist 2002; 42(5): 643–52.

60. Chappell NL. Implications of shifting health care policy for caregiving in Canada. J Aging Social Policy 1993; 5: 39–55.

Index

Page numbers in *italics* refer to tables and figures.

acetylcholine (ACh) 64, *66*
acetylcholinesterase inhibitors (AChEIs) 107–8
  clinical use 93, *93*, 110, *110*
  development 22
  pharmacology 108–10
    chemical structures *23*, *108*
    effects on specific measures *109*
    mechanism of action *108*
AD *see* Alzheimer's disease (AD)
AD Anti-Inflammatory Prevention Trial (ADAPT) *89*, 93
age
  as AD risk factor 34
  and incidence of dementia 29, 31, *33*, *34*
  and prevalence of dementia 28, *28*, *29*
agitation management 114
alcohol consumption and AD prevention 97
alpha-tocopherol *see* vitamin E
aluminium exposure and AD risk 97, *98*
Alzheimer, Alois *1*, 6–13, *8*, *9*, *10*
Alzheimer's disease (AD)
  diagnosis *see* diagnosis of AD and dementia
  future research
    biomarkers 54–5, *55*, 126–7
    genomics and proteomics 125–6, *126*
    neuroimaging 127–9, *128*, *129*
  future societal/economic implications 133–4, *133*, *134*
  incidence 29, 31, *34*
  pathophysiology 59–69
  potential biomarkers 54–5, *55*, 126–7
  prevalence 28–9, *31*, *32*
    effect of delayed disease onset 32–3, *35*, *85*
  prevention 83–103
  rate of cognitive decline and mortality 32, *34*
  risk factors *33*
    age 34
    educational level 35–6, *35*, 98
    ethnicity 36, *36*
    family history *35*, 36, *36*
    gender 34–5, *35*
    genetic *see* genetics and AD
  survival after diagnosis 31–2, *34*

symptom progression 105–6, *105*
vascular pathology *90*
see also historical concepts of AD and dementia; treatment of AD
Alzheimer's Disease Assessment Scale-Cognitive Subscale (ADAS-cog) 106
Alzheimer's Disease Cooperative Study-Activities of Daily Living (ADCS-ADL) 107
Alzheimer's Disease Neuroimaging Initiative (ADNI) 127
amentia 5
amyloid 72
amyloid antiaggregants 118–19, 129–30
amyloid beta (Aβ) protein
  as AD biomarker 54, *55*, 126–7
  in AD pathogenesis 80
  neurotoxicity 19, *20*
  see also senile plaques (SPs)
amyloid beta (Aβ) vaccination
  clinical trial results 117, *118*
  meningoencephalitis in human subjects 118, *118*, *119*
  mouse studies 117, *117*, 131, *132*
  peptide structure of initial vaccine *132*
amyloid cascade hypothesis 17, 19, *19*, *20*, 80
amyloid precursor protein (APP) 61–2, *62*, *66*, 72, *72*
amyloid precursor protein (APP) gene mutations 36, *37*, 62–3
antiaggregants 118–19, 129–30
antibiotic therapy 120
antidepressant therapy 114, *115–16*
antihypertensive therapy 90–1, *91*
anti-inflammatory agents 92–3, *92*, 120, 132–3
antioxidants 94, 119, *120*, 132
antipsychotics 114
apathy management 113–14, *114*
apolipoprotein E (ApoE)
  ApoE e4 and AD risk 17, 36, *37*, 38, 63–4
  functions 63, *65*
  isoforms *37*, 63, *64*
  role in AD *65*
Aristotle 2, *3*
assessment of AD symptoms 106–7, *107*

atorvastatin 120–1, *121*
Auguste D case 9–13, *12*

Babes, Victor 5, 7
Bacon, Roger 2, *4*
β-sheet breakers 129–30
Bielschowsky, Max 9, *11*
Binswanger, Otto 5, 7
biomarkers for AD 54–5, *55*, 126–7
Blocq, Paul 5
blood, AD biomarkers in 54–5, *55*
blood pressure and AD/dementia 66, *67*, 86–7, 90, *91*
body weight and risk of dementia 92
brain plasticity 85
brain volume loss 49–50
Bronx aging study *95*, *96*
burned-out senile plaques 72, *73*

Camelford incident *98*
Canadian Study of Health and Aging 97
candesartan *89*, 90
carbamazepine 114
caspase inhibitors 132
celecoxib *89*, 93
CEP 1347 131
cerebral amyloid angiopathy (CAA) 66, 75–6, *79*
cerebral atrophy 49–50, *50*, 71, *72*
cerebral cortex, architectonic representation *59*
Cerebri Anatome: Cui Accessit Nervorum Descriptio et Usus (Willis) 2
cerebrolysin 121
cerebrospinal fluid AD biomarkers 54, *55*, 126–7
chelating agents 119, 130
cholesterol and AD 64, 91, 120–1, *121*
cholinergic hypothesis of AD 16, *17*
cholinergic system *130*
cholinesterase inhibitors *see* acetylcholinesterase inhibitors (AChEIs)
chromosome 21 16, 63
citalopram *115*, *116*
Clinician's Interview-Based Impression of Change scale (CIBIC-Plus) 106
clioquinol 119, 130
clomipramine *115*
coenzyme Q10 132
cognitive activities and AD prevention 94–6, *95*, *96*, *97*
cognitive assessment 106
cognitively impaired not demented (CIND) 35, *35*
cognitive reserve hypothesis 36, 85, *86*
computed tomography (CT) 19, *21*, 48, *48*
corticobasal degeneration (CBD) 46–7
'cotton-wool' plaques 77, *81*
Creutzfeld–Jacob disease (CJD) 47–8
Cullen, William 2, *4*
curcumin 132
cystatin 3 *126*

dementia
  19th Century causes *6*
  differential diagnosis 45–8, *46*
  early onset 28, *32*, 36

incidence studies 29, 31, *33*, *34*
mixed *41*, 77–8
prevalence studies 27–9, *28*, *29*, *31*, *41*
survival after diagnosis 31–2, *34*
treatable causes 44
see also Alzheimer's disease (AD); historical concepts of AD and dementia
dementia with Lewy bodies (DLB) *41*, 47, 78
depression management 114, *115–16*
Des Maladies Mentales (Esquirol) 5
diabetes mellitus 91
diagnosis of AD and dementia 41–57
  AD diagnostic criteria 20, 22, 41–4, 77, *80*
    DSM-IV TR 41, *42*, *43–4*, *45*
    ICD-10 41, *43–4*
    NINCDS-ADRDA 41, *42–3*, *43–4*, *45*
    sensitivity and specificity *45*
    similarities and differences *43–4*
  clinical diagnosis of AD 44–5
  differential diagnosis of dementia 45–8, *46*
  neuroimaging approaches 48
    functional 50–3, *50*, *51*, *52*, *53*, *54*
    structural 48–50, *48*, *49*, *50*
  neuropathologic 77, *80*
  potential AD biomarkers 54–5, *55*, 126–7
Diagnostic and Statistical Manual of Mental Disorders, 4th edition, text revision (DSM-IV-TR) criteria for AD 41, *42*, *43–4*, *45*
dietary fat intake and AD 92
diffuse senile plaques 72–3, *73*
diffusion tensor imaging (DTI) 53, *54*
Disability Assessment for Dementia (DAD) 107
divalproex sodium 114
donepezil
  chemical structure *23*, *108*
  combined with memantine 110, *113*
  dosage and titration *110*
  effect on specific measures *109*
  mechanism of action 108, *108*
  treatment of MCI 93, *93*
Down's syndrome (DS) 16, *18*, 63

early onset dementia 28, *32*, 36
economic and societal implications of AD 133–4, *133*, *134*
education and AD risk 35–6, *35*, 98
electromagnetic radiation and AD risk 97–8
electron microscopy (EM), early studies of AD pathology 15, *15*
enalapril *89*
entorhinal cortex 50, *50*
epidemiology of AD and dementia 27–40
  incidence studies 29, 31, *33*, *34*
  prevalence studies
    dementia subtypes 28–9, *31*, *32*
    effect of delaying AD onset 32–3, *35*, *84*
    worldwide 27–8, *28*, *29*, *31*
  risk factors for AD 33–8, *35*, *36*, *37*
  survival after diagnosis 31–2, *34*
episodic memory 45
Esquirol, Jean Etienne 5, *6*
estrogen 87, *89*, 92, 133

ethnicity and AD risk 36, *36*
executive dysfunction 45

familial AD 77, 125, *126*
family history and AD risk *35*, 36, *36*
fat intake and AD 92
[18F]FDDNP (fluorine-18-labelled FDDNP) 20, 50–1, *52*, 128
fish consumption and risk of dementia 92
fluoxetine *115*
R-flurbiprofen 129
flurodeoxyglucose-PET (FDG-PET) 19–20, 50, *51*, *52*, 127, *128*
folate 93–4, *94*
FPF-1070 (cerebrolysin) 121
frontotemporal degeneration/dementia (FTD) 28, *31*, *41*, 45–6
frontotemporal dementia-motor neuron disease (FTD-MND) 47
frontotemporal lobular degeneration (FTD; Pick complex) 45–7
functional assessment 107
functional imaging 50–3, *50*, *51*, *52*, *53*, *54*

galantamine
    chemical structure *23*, *108*
    dosage and titration *110*
    effect on specific measures *109*
    mechanism of action 108, *109*
Galen 2, *3*
Geisenheimer, Nathalie (married Dr Alzheimer) 7, *8*
GEMS trial *89*
gender and AD risk 34–5, *35*
genetics and AD 36–8, *37*, 62–4, *64*
    early studies 16–17, *18*
    future research 125, *126*
genomics 125, *126*
Ginkgo biloba *89*, 94
glitazones (thiazolidenediones) 91
global assessment 106
glucose metabolism, neuroimaging 50, *51*, *52*
glutamate 22, *24*, 111
glutamate antagonism *see* memantine
glutaminergic basis of AD therapy 22, *24*
glycogen synthase kinase (GSK) inhibitors 131–2
Golgi, Camillo 9, *11*
granulovacuolar degeneration (GVD) 76, *79*
Greco-Roman concepts of dementia 1–2, *3*
GUIDAGE trial *89*

head injury and AD risk 98
health promotion 98–100, *99*, *100*
Heart Outcome Prevention Evaluations (HOPE) study 90, *91*
hippocampal atrophy *49*, 72
Hippocrates 2, *3*
Hirano bodies 77, *79*
historical concepts of AD and dementia 1–26
    origins of dementia
        Greco-Roman period 1–2
        Middle Ages 2, *4*

17th–19th centuries 2, 3–5, *4*, *5*, 6, 7
20th century
    Alois Alzheimer *1*, 6–13, *8*, *9*, *10*
    1910–30 13
    1930–1980 13–16, *15*, *16*
    1980–present
        amyloid cascade hypothesis 17, 19, *19*, *20*
        diagnostic criteria 20, 22
        genetics 16–17, *18*
        neuroimaging 19–20, *21*
        treatment 22–4, *23*, *24*
homocysteine 93–4, *94*
hormonal treatment, luteinizing hormone 133
hormone replacement therapy (HRT) 87, *89*, 92, 133
hydrochlorothiazide *89*
hypertension and AD 66, *67*, 86–7, 90, *91*

imipramine *115*
incidence 27
inflammation in AD pathogenesis 62, *63*, 77
insulin-degrading enzyme *126*
International Classification of Diseases 10th Revision (ICD-10) criteria for AD *41*, *43–4*
intravenous immunoglobulin (IVIg) 119
ischemia and AD 64, 66
isoprostanes 55

Johann F case 13, *14*
cJun N-terminal kinase (JNK) 131

Kraepelin, Emil 7, *9–10*, 13
Kungsholmen Project 93, 98

leisure activities and AD prevention 94–6, *95*, *96*
length bias 31
lifestyle and AD prevention 94–7, *95*, *96*, *97*
lithium 132
London Practice of Physick (Willis) 2
long-term potentiation (LTP) 22
luteinizing hormone 133
LY450139 dihydrate 129

magnetic resonance imaging (MRI)
    development 19
    diffusion tensor imaging (DTI) 53, *54*
    functional MRI (fMRI) 19, *21*, 52, *53*, 127, *128*
    future directions 127, *128*
    magnetic resonance spectroscopy (MRS) 51–2, *53*
    magnetization transfer imaging (MTI) 52–3
    use in AD diagnosis 48–50, *49*, *50*
maprotiline *115*
Marinescu, Gheorghe 5, 7
memantine
    chemical structure *24*, *110*
    combined with donepezil 111, *113*
    dosage and titration *110*
    effects in AD 111, *112*
    mechanism of action 22, 110, *111*
    side effects 111
memory deficits 45
meningoencephalitis after Aβ vaccination 117–18, *118*, *119*

methionine–homocysteine–folate–B12 cycle *94*
Methods of Preventing the Appearance of Senility (Bacon) 2
mild cognitive impairment (MCI) 49–50, *50*, 83, 93
miliary sclerosis 5
mixed dementia *41*, 77–8
moclobemide *115*
motor neuron disease (MND) 47
multi-infarct dementia (MID) 16
Multiple Outcomes of Raloxifene Evaluation (MORE)
    study 92

N-acetylaspartate (NAA) 52, *53*
naproxen *89*, 93
National Institute of Neurological and Communicative
    Disorders and Stroke-Alzheimer's Disease and
    Related Disorders Association (NINCDS-ADRDA)
    criteria for AD 41, *42–3, 43–4, 45*
nerve growth factor (NGF) 133
neural stem cells in adult human brain *85*
neuritic senile plaques 72, *73, 73, 74*
neurofibrillary tangles (NFTs) *59*
   and AD pathogenesis 78
   conditions in which they occur 60
   early ultrastructural studies 15, *15*
   formation 60–1, *60, 61*
   from Auguste D *12*
   microscopic appearance 75, *76*
   in non-demented individuals 77
   progressive accumulation 75, *78*
   regional distribution 75, *75*
   ultrastructure of paired helical filaments 75, 77
neuroimaging
   development 19–20, *21*
   functional 50–3, *50, 51, 52, 53, 54*
   future directions 127–9, *128, 129*
   structural 48–50, *48, 49, 50*
neuropathology 71–81
   familial AD 77
   gross pathology 71, *72*
   microscopic pathology *72*
     cerebral amyloid angiopathy 66, 75–6, *79*
     chronic inflammation 77
     granulovacuolar degeneration 76, *79*
     Hirano bodies 77, *79*
     neuropil threads 75, *76*
     see also neurofibrillary tangles (NFTs); senile plaques
      (SPs)
   mixed dementia 77–8
   non-demented elderly individuals 77, *79*
   pathogenesis of AD 78, 80–1
   pathologic AD diagnostic criteria 77, *80*
neuropil threads 75, *76*
Neuropsychiatric Inventory (NPI) 107
neuropsychiatric symptoms
   assessment 106–7, *107*
   management 111–13, *114*
     apathy 113–14
     depression 114, *115–16*
     psychosis and agitation 114
neurotransmitter deficits in AD 64
neurotropic factors 121–2, 133

Nissl, Franz 6–7, *9–10*
nitrendipine 89, 90, *91*
non-steroidal anti-inflammatory drugs (NSAIDs) 92–3, *92*,
    120, 132
normal-pressure hydrocephalus (NPH) 47
Nun study 90
Nurses' Health Study 96, 98

obesity and risk of dementia 92
occupation and AD risk 98
omega-3 polyunsaturated fatty acids 92
ONO-2506 133

paired helical filaments (PHFs) 15, *15*, 75, 77
Parkinson disease dementia (PDD) 47
pathophysiology of AD 59–69
   and architectonic evolution of brain 59, *59*
   effects of ischemia 64, 66
   evidence for inflammatory mechanisms 62, *63*
   histopathology 59–62, *59, 60, 61, 62*
     see also neurofibrillary tangles (NFTs); senile plaques
     (SPs)
   neurotransmitter deficits 64
   overview *130*
   role of cholesterol 64, 120–1
   see also genetics and AD
perindropril 90, *91*
Perindropril Protection Against Recurrent Stroke
    (PROGRESS) study 90, *91*
Perusini, Gaetano 13
physical activity and AD prevention 95, 96–7, *96, 97*
physostigmine 22, *23*, 108, *108*
Pick complex (frontotemporal lobular degeneration; FTD)
    45–7
Pinel, Philippe 4–5, *5*
Pittsburgh compound B (PIB) 20, 50–1, 128, *129*
plasticity 85
positron emission tomography (PET) 19–20, *21*, 50–1, *51, 52*
   future directions 129–31, *128, 129*
PREADVISE trial *89*
PREPARE trial *89*
presenilin gene mutations 17, 36, *37*, 63, *64*
prevalence 27
prevention of AD 83–103
   biological plausibility 85, *86*
   candidate interventions
     lifestyle 94–7, *95, 96, 97*
     pharmacologic 92–3, *92, 93*
     vascular risk factor targeting 90–2, *90, 91*
     vitamins/complementary medications 93–4, *94*
     others 97–8
   evidence
     primary prevention RCTs 88–90, *89*
     risk factor information from observational studies 87–8,
      87, 88
   modifiable protective factors *87*
   modifiable risk factors *87*
   public policy/health promotion 98–100, *99, 100*
   spectrum of interventions 83, *84*
   timing 86–7, *86*
primitive neuritic senile plaques 72, *73*

Progressive Deterioration Scale (PDS) 107
progressive supranuclear palsy (PSP) 47
proteomics 126
psychosis management 114
Pythagoras 1–2, *3*

raloxifene 92
ramipril 90, *91*
REM sleep behavioral disorder 47
R-flurbiprofen 129
rifampicin 120
rivastigmine
   brain metabolic effects in AD *51*
   chemical structure *23*, *108*
   dosage and titration *110*
   effect on specific measures *109*
   mechanism of action 108, *109*

secretases 17, *18*, 62
secretase inhibitors 117, 129
selenium *89*
semantic memory 45
senile plaques (SPs)
   and AD pathogenesis 78, 80
   composition 71–2, *73*
   distribution in AD 73, 75, *75*
   formation 61–2, *62*
   from Auguste D *12*
   morphologic types 61, 72–3, *73*, *74*
   in non-demented individuals 77, *79*
sertraline *115*, *116*
Severe Impairment Battery (SIB) 106
single photon emission CT (SPECT) 19, *21*, *50*, 51, 129
smoking and AD prevention 97
social/leisure activities and AD prevention 94–6, *95*, *96*
societal and economic implications of AD 133–4, *133*, *134*
statins 91, 120–1, *121*, 130–1
stress kinase signaling inhibitors 131
stroke 90–1
Study on Cognition and Prognosis in the Elderly (SCOPE) *89*, 90
symptom evaluation in AD 106–7, *107*
symptom progression in AD 105–6, *105*
Systolic Hypertension in Europe (SYST-EUR) trial *89*, 90, *91*

tacrine *23*, 108, *108*
tau gene mutations 17

tau phosphorylation inhibitors 131–2
tau protein
   in AD 60–1, *60*, *61*
   as AD biomarker 54, *55*, 127
   binding to microtubules 60
tetracycline 120
thiazolidenediones (glitazones) 91
tramiprosate 118, 130
Treatise on Insanity (Pinel) 4
treatment of AD 22–4, 105–24
   disease-modification strategies 115, *117*, *131*
      amyloid antiaggregants 118–19, 129–30
      antibiotics 120
      anti-inflammatory agents 92–3, *92*, 120, 132–3
      antioxidants 94, 119, *120*, 132
      caspase inhibitors 132
      cholesterol-lowering agents 91, 120–1, *121*, 130–1
      hormonal treatment 133
      neurotropic factors 121–2, 133
      secretase modulation 117, 129
      stress kinase signaling inhibitors 131
      tau phosphorylation inhibitors 131–2
      see also amyloid beta (Aβ) vaccination
   symptomatic treatments 129
      neuropsychiatric symptoms 111–13, 114, *114*
      symptom evaluation 106–7, *107*
      target symptoms 105–6, *105*
      see also acetylcholinesterase inhibitors (AChEIs); memantine
   treatment effects *84*
trisomy 21 (Down's syndrome; DS) 16, *18*, 63

vaccination *see* amyloid beta (Aβ) vaccination
valproate 132
vascular dementia (VaD) 16, 29, *33*, 34, *35*, 47
vascular risk factors as targets for AD prevention 90–2, *90*, *91*
Virchow, Rudolf 5, 7
vitamin B12 93, *94*
vitamin C 94
vitamin E *89*, 94, 119, *120*, 132

Washington Heights–Inwood aging project *95*
weight and risk of dementia 92
WHO world regions *30*
Wilks, Sir Samuel 5, 7
Willis, Thomas 2, *4*
Women's Health Initiative Study (WHIMS) *89*, 92
Women Who Walk Study 96

Printed and bound by CPI Group (UK) Ltd, Croydon, CR0 4YY

23/10/2024

01778226-0020